Ovarian Cancer

This volume is the first of a new series dedicated to the historical developments in topics that are central to gynecological cancers. The six essays on ovarian cancer included here provide context from the perspective of experts in the field, illustrating what is required for the development and realization of medical innovation: (i) time consuming, decades-long basic research of the tumor genome and cancer cell biology, which may then set the basis for dramatic accelerations of recent therapeutic options; and (ii) the diligent assessment and fine-tuning of surgical techniques and concepts of patient prehabilitation and rehabilitation.

Series Title: Developments in Gynecologic Oncology

Ovarian Cancer

Edited by

Malte Renz, MD PhD

Gynecologic Oncologist,
Charité Universitätsmedizin Berlin,
Germany

CRC Press
Taylor & Francis Group
Boca Raton London New York

CRC Press is an imprint of the
Taylor & Francis Group, an **informa** business

First edition published 2026
by CRC Press
2385 NW Executive Center Drive, Suite 320, Boca Raton FL 33431

and by CRC Press
4 Park Square, Milton Park, Abingdon, Oxon, OX14 4RN

CRC Press is an imprint of Taylor & Francis Group, LLC

© 2026 selection and editorial matter, Malte Renz; individual chapters, the contributors

ISBN: 978-1-032-32033-5 (hbk)
ISBN: 978-1-032-32034-2 (pbk)
ISBN: 978-1-003-31247-5 (ebk)

DOI: 10.1201/9781003312475

Typeset in Times
by SPi Technologies India Pvt Ltd (Straive)

Contents

Preface   vi
Contributors   viii

1 **Early Detection of Ovarian Cancer: An Update**   1
  Chae Young Han, Zhen Lu, Karen H. Lu, Jacob S. Bedia,
  Anna Lokshin, Karen S. Anderson, Charles W. Drescher,
  Steven Skates, and Robert C. Bast Jr.

2 **History of Cytoreductive Surgery in Ovarian Cancer**
  Treatment   26
  Alex A. Francoeur, Robert Bristow, and Jill Tseng

3 **Hereditary Breast and Ovarian Cancer: A Historical**
  Perspective   47
  Payal D. Shah and Susan M. Domchek

4 **History of PARP Inhibitors**   68
  Malte Renz and Jonathan S. Berek

5 **History and Current Role of Immunotherapy in Ovarian**
  Cancer Treatment   84
  Stephanie Chow and Oliver Dorigo

6 **The History and Current Role of Perioperative Care and**
  Prehabilitation in Ovarian Cancer   101
  Marlene Misu Lee and Jalid Sehouli

Index   123

Preface

Two things are necessary for our work: tireless perseverance and the willingness to throw away something you have put a lot of time and effort into.

Albert Einstein (1879–1955)

With this preface to *Ovarian Cancer* – Volume 1 in a series on developments in cancers from CRC Press – I am delighted to introduce an entirely new series of essays dedicated to the historical developments of topics that are central to gynecological cancers. We start the book series with six essays on ovarian cancer. These essays are intended to shed light on historic developments and provide context to central topics in ovarian cancer from the perspective of experts in the field. Beyond historical developments in medicine, this first collection of essays illustrates what is required for the development and realization of medical innovation: (i) time consuming, decades-long basic research of the tumor genome and cancer cell biology which may then set the basis for dramatic accelerations of recent therapeutic options; and (ii) the diligent assessment and fine-tuning of surgical techniques and concepts of patient prehabilitation and rehabilitation.

The essays collected here address the following aspects of ovarian cancer: screening, surgical treatment, prehabilitation and rehabilitation, genetic predisposition, targeted therapy exemplified by PARP inhibitors, and immunotherapy. Robert Bast et al. describe the efforts to establish efficient screening programs for ovarian cancer since the discovery of the tumor marker Ca125 by Dr. Bast. Robert Bristow et al. provide the available evidence for cytoreductive or debulking surgeries in ovarian cancer. Susan Domchek et al. give an account of the historical developments of hereditary breast and ovarian cancer syndrome. Jonathan Berek et al. recount breakthroughs and limitations in targeted therapy leading to PARP-inhibitor use. Oliver Dorigo et al. outline recent immunotherapy developments. Finally, Jalid Sehouli and co-workers lay out plans for prehabilitation and rehabilitation programs that include and expand existing ERAS programs.

I hope that these essays provide pearls of knowledge and context for those who aim to continuously study gynecologic oncology. These essays are synopses of the developments over time in a specific field, just like short monographs. This essay series is meant for those who study gynecologic oncology, clinical fellows and experienced physicians as well as clinical and basic researchers. They may provide an improved understanding and give a glimpse into the temporary and at times provisional nature of medical knowledge and its constant flux. And maybe the insights provided here, including the insights into the temporality of research and clinical achievements, will inspire new avenues and developments in ovarian cancer.

Malte Renz

Contributors

Karen S. Anderson
Biodesign Institute
Arizona State University
Tempe, Arizona

Robert C. Bast, Jr.
Department of Experimental
 Therapeutics
University of Texas M.D. Anderson
 Cancer Center
Houston, Texas

Jacob S. Bedia
Biostatistics Center
Massachusetts General Hospital
Boston, Massachusetts

Jonathan S. Berek
Division of Gynecology Stanford
 Cancer Institute
Stanford, California

Robert Bristow
Department of Gynecologic
 Oncology
University of California Irvine
Orange, California

Stephanie Chow
Department of Obstetrics and
 Gynecology
Division of Gynecologic Oncology
Stanford Cancer Institute
Stanford, California

Susan M. Domchek
Perelman School of Medicine at the
 University of Pennsylvania
Basser Center for BRCA
Abramson Cancer Center
University of Pennsylvania
Philadelphia, Pennsylvania

Oliver Dorigo
Department of Obstetrics and
 Gynecology
Division of Gynecologic
 Oncology
Stanford Cancer Institute
Stanford, California

Charles W. Drescher
Gynecologic Oncology
Fred Hutchinson Cancer Research
 Center
Seattle, Washington

Alex A. Francoeur
Department of Gynecologic
 Oncology
University of California Irvine
Orange, California

Chae Young Han
Department of Experimental
 Therapeutics
University of Texas M.D. Anderson
 Cancer Center
Houston, Texas

Marlene Misu Lee
Department of Gynecology with
  Center for Oncological Surgery
Charité – Universitätsmedizin Berlin
Berlin, Germany

Zhen Lu
Department of Experimental
  Therapeutics
University of Texas M.D. Anderson
  Cancer Center
Houston, Texas

Karen H. Lu
Moffit Cancer Center
Tampa, Florida

Anna Lokshin
Department of Obstetrics and
  Gynecology
University of Pittsburgh School of
  Medicine
Pittsburgh, Pennsylvania

Malte Renz
Department of Gynecology with
  Center for Oncological Surgery
Charité – Universitätsmedizin Berlin
Berlin, Germany

Jalid Sehouli
Department of Gynecology with
  Center for Oncological Surgery
Charité – Universitätsmedizin Berlin
Berlin, Germany

Payal D. Shah
Perelman School of Medicine at the
  University of Pennsylvania
Basser Center for BRCA
Abramson Cancer Center
University of Pennsylvania
Philadelphia, Pennsylvania

Steven Skates
Biostatistics Center
Massachusetts General Hospital
Boston, Massachusetts

Jill Tseng
Department of Gynecologic
  Oncology
University of California Irvine
Orange, California

Early Detection of Ovarian Cancer

An Update

1

Chae Young Han, Zhen Lu, Karen H. Lu,
Jacob S. Bedia, Anna Lokshin, Karen
S. Anderson, Charles W. Drescher,
Steven Skates, and Robert C. Bast Jr.

1.1 BACKGROUND

This year in the United States 19,710 women will develop ovarian cancer and 13,270 will die from the disease (1). Worldwide, more than 300,000 women are afflicted annually (2). Poor outcomes for women with ovarian cancer relate to detection of the disease at a late stage (III, IV) in more than 70% of cases and to the persistence of drug-resistant cancer cells after primary surgery and chemotherapy, often in a dormant state on the surface of the peritoneal cavity. Earlier detection of ovarian cancer could improve clinical outcomes. When limited to the ovaries at diagnosis (Stage I), 93% of ovarian cancer patients survive 5 years (3). Even when disease has spread to the pelvis (Stage II),

DOI: 10.1201/9781003312475-1

5-year survival exceeds 70%. By contrast, when cancer has metastasized to the abdominal cavity (Stage III) or into the parenchyma of the liver or above the diaphragm (Stage IV), 5-year survival slips to 31%. At present less than 30% of ovarian cancers are diagnosed in early stage (I–II). Computer models indicate that mortality could be reduced by 10–30% if a greater fraction of ovarian cancers were diagnosed in early stage (4), provided that a stage shift is associated with decreased mortality. As the prevalence of ovarian cancer is 1 in 2,500 for postmenopausal women at average risk for the disease, a successful screening strategy must have both high sensitivity and very high specificity. To achieve an adequate positive predictive value (PPV) of 10% with no more than 10 operations per ovarian cancer detected requires a sensitivity of $\geq 75\%$ for asymptomatic disease and a specificity $> 99.6\%$ (5). This performance level of such a high specificity is difficult to achieve, particularly with a single screening modality.

1.2 DISCOVERY AND DEVELOPMENT OF CA125

Attempts to detect ovarian cancer at an earlier stage have used transvaginal ultrasound (TVS) and the blood biomarker CA125. The discovery of CA125 is a study in serendipity. In the early 1970's, the tuberculosis vaccine *Bacillus calmette* Guerin (BCG), an attenuated strain of bovine tubercle bacillus, was used to treat patients with melanoma, where intratumoral injection of BCG produced intense granulomatous inflammation and regression of cutaneous melanoma metastases (6, 7). In some patients, non-injected lesions regressed consistent with the induction of systemic immunity. Rapp and Zbar obtained formal evidence for the immune adjuvant activity of BCG using a guinea pig hepatoma model where intratumoral injection of BCG cured subcutaneous transplants and lymph node metastases, rendering animals specifically immune to re-challenge (8). Clinical application of BCG was extended to intravesical administration to treat superficial bladder cancers (6, 7).

As ovarian cancer grows on the peritoneal surface, intraperitoneal administration of BCG might eliminate small volumes of residual disease that remained after cytoreductive surgery and combination chemotherapy. Risk of progressive infection, however, discouraged use of living BCG for intraperitoneal therapy. Heat-killed *Corynebacterium parvum* provided similar antitumor activity after intraperitoneal injection without the risk of infection. Knapp and colleagues developed a syngeneic murine ovarian cancer transplant model, where cancer cells could grow intraperitoneally, block diaphragmatic lymphatics and produce ascites, resembling human ovarian cancer (9). Treatment with rabbit antibodies against the murine ovarian cancer prolonged survival. Addition of *C. parvum* proved synergistic, enhancing median survival and producing long term survivors (9). The synergistic effect of antibody and *C. parvum* related to antibody dependent cell mediated cytotoxicity (ADCC) where the *C. parvum* attracted and activated immune effectors that could bind to and kill antibody-coated cancer cells (10).

Translating this model to the clinic, intraperitoneal administration of *C. parvum* through a dialysis catheter produced a 32% objective response rate in patients with small volumes of recurrent ovarian cancer with two CR's lasting 5 and 12 months (11). Importantly, intraperitoneal *C. Parvum* attracted and activated effectors for ADCC, paralleling results in the murine model.

To prepare adequate amounts of specific antibody, the then new technology developed by Kohler and Milstein was used to develop the first monoclonal antibodies reactive with human ovarian cancer. The 125th promising clone (OC125) bound to ovarian cancer cell lines, but not to a B lymphocyte cell line from the same patient (12).

The antigen recognized by OC125, designated Cancer Antigen 125 (CA125), was expressed by 80% of ovarian cancers, suggesting that a large fraction of patients might benefit from OC125 treatment. CA125 was, however, shed from the cancer cell surface. Shed antigen could neutralize the effect of the OC125 antibody before it bound to ovarian cancer cells, preventing enhanced immunotherapy with *C. parvum*. Shed antigen might provide a biomarker for disease burden.

CA125 was found to be a mucin (MUC16) ranging in molecular weight to 5 million Daltons (13). For ovarian cancers that express CA125, up to a million copies are found on the surface of each cancer cell. CA125 is cleaved and shed from the cancer cell surface by proteolysis and finds its way to the bloodstream. The presence of > 60 identical 40 KD tandem repeats on CA125's extracellular domain facilitated the development of a homologous double determinant immunoassay using the OC125 antibody. Given multiple identical epitopes on each CA125 molecule, the same OC125 antibody could be used to trap antigen on a bead and to detect antigen that had been trapped (14). O'Brian subsequently developed the M11 antibody against a distinct epitope on MUC16, permitting the development of a heterologous double determinant assay with less day-to-day variation using this assay (15), CA125 levels are elevated in more than 80% of ovarian cancers. CA125 tracks response to treatment and recurrence in more than 70% of patients, rising 4 months before signs and symptoms of recurrent disease (16). In 1987 CA125 was approved by the US FDA for detection of persistent disease after primary surgery and chemotherapy. In addition to monitoring response to treatment and detecting persistent or recurrent disease, CA125 has been incorporated into the ROMA and

OVERA algorithms to identify patients with a pelvic mass who would benefit from referral to a gynecologic oncologist (17, 18).

1.3 SCREENING WOMEN AT AVERAGE RISK

1.3.1 Single Modality Screening with CA125 or Transvaginal Sonography (TVS)

Attempts to detect ovarian cancer in early stage have generally used two approaches – the blood biomarker CA125 (12, 14, 15) or transvaginal sonography (TVS) (19, 20). In large randomized studies, neither serum CA125 nor TVS have achieved adequate sensitivity or specificity for early detection of ovarian cancer (21). In the Prostate, Lung, Colon, and Ovary (PLCO) Cancer Screening Trial, 78,216 postmenopausal women were randomized to be screened annually with CA125 for 6 years and TVS for 4 years or to receive conventional care (22). Both groups were followed for a median of 14 years (22). The protocol provided results of both tests to the patient and the health care provider for subsequent undefined management. Detection with either CA125 or TVS produced a low PPV of 1.2%. Detection with an elevated CA125 (> 35 U/mL) alone or abnormal TVS alone produced only modest PPVs of 3.7% and 1% respectively. When both tests were abnormal, the PPV rose to 23.5%, but 80% of the ovarian cancer cases would have been missed.

Another large trial in Japan randomized asymptomatic postmenopausal women to annual screening with TVS and CA125 (41,688) or to conventional care (40,799) (23). Screening was associated with a higher fraction of cases in stage I (63%) than with conventional care (38%), but this difference failed to reach statistical significance (P = 0.23).

1.3.2 Two Stage Screening Strategies with CA125 Followed by TVS

Two-stage strategies have been developed using rising CA125 to trigger TVS in a small fraction of women. In patients with ovarian cancer, CA125 rises over time above each woman's individual CA125 baseline reflecting growth of the cancer. CA125 can be elevated (> 35 U/mL) by benign conditions but generally

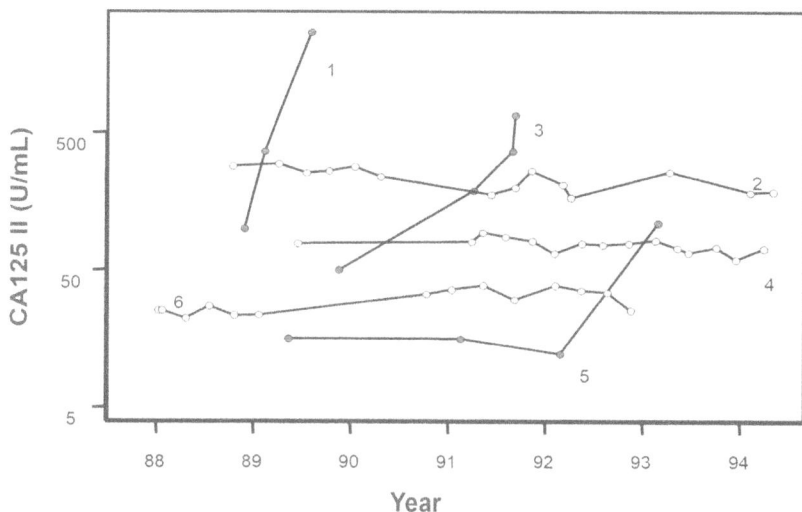

FIGURE 1.1 Serial pattern of CA125 levels in 6 women from a UK study prospective trial of 22,000 postmenopausal women. CA125 values for 3 women with occult ovarian cancer (filled circles) and 3 women without ovarian cancer (open circles). (From Ref. 21 with permission.)

does not rise over time as benign lesions grow slowly, if at all (Figure 1.1). To quantify these trends, Steven Skates developed a Bayesian Risk of Ovarian Cancer Algorithm (ROCA) to analyze serial CA125 values (24, 25) to calculate the probability of the CA125 having an exponential increase above a baseline due to a tumor doubling over time rather than a background CA125 fluctuation. The ROCA algorithm estimates the risk of actually having undetected ovarian cancer based on the profile of CA125 values for a woman over time. If the risk based on a significantly rising CA125 is elevated, the screen prompts TVS and abnormal imaging triggers referral to a gynecologic oncologist to determine whether surgery should be undertaken (Figure 1.2). Based on ROCA scores, participants can be triaged to groups with normal, intermediate and high risk. When risk is normal (< 1:2000), women return in one year for an annual CA125 determination. When risk is elevated (> 1:500), TVS is carried out and the participant referred to a gynecologic oncologist for possible surgery based on TVS. If risk is intermediate (< 1:500 and > 1:2,000), CA125 measurement is repeated in 3 months, risk re-calculated, and the participant re-triaged to return in 9 months or to undergo TVS.

Using this two-stage approach can enhance both specificity and sensitivity. Referral of only 2% of participants to TVS achieves a specificity of 98%. Specificity is further improved by TVS. The sequential application of the two

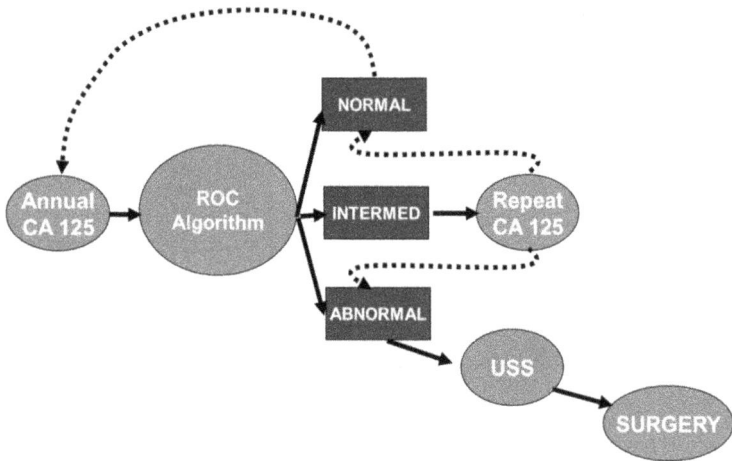

FIGURE 1.2   Two-stage screening strategy using the risk of ovarian cancer algorithm (ROCA). (From Ref. 21 with permission.)

tests achieves a very high specificity of 99.8%. Some ovarian cancer patients experience a rapid rise in CA125 within 12 months (Figure 1.3), while others exhibit a more gradual rise in CA125, detecting ovarian cancer while CA125 is still within normal limits (< 35 U/mL). Detection of ovarian cancer while CA125 is in the normal range can enhance sensitivity.

1.3.3 Two Major ROCA–driven Ovarian Cancer Screening Trials

The ROCA–driven two-stage strategy has been evaluated in two major trials: the United Kingdom Collaborative Trial of Ovarian Cancer Screening (UKCTOCS) (26–29) and the Normal Risk Ovarian Cancer Screening Study (NROSS) in the United States (30, 31). Both have tested the same two-stage multi-modality screening (MMS) strategy using the ROCA to estimate risk associated with rising CA125 followed by TVS in a small fraction of subjects.

In the UKCTOCS, > 200,000 postmenopausal women at average risk were randomly assigned to one of three groups: 1) a control group (101,314) followed through the national tumor registry (26); 2) annual screening with TVS (50,623) for 7 to 11 years; or 3) multimodal screening (50,640) using annual CA125 analyzed with the ROCA followed by TVS in 2% of subjects per year for 7–11 years. In an initial analysis, multimodality screening reduced mortality by 20% in a prespecified subgroup that excluded prevalent cases

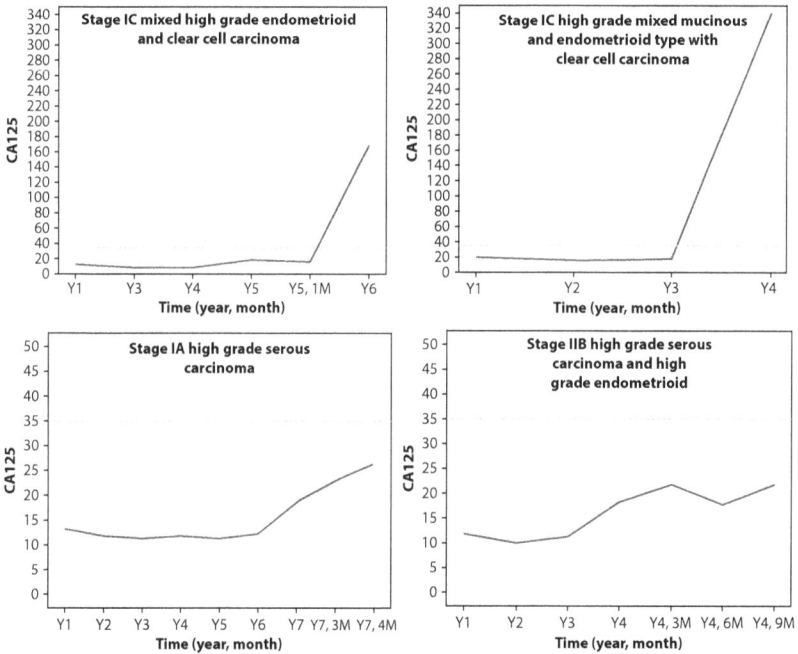

FIGURE 1.3 Serial CA125 values for 4 patients with early stage ovarian cancer detected on the NROSS trial. (a) stage IC mixed grade endometrioid and clear cell carcinoma; (b) stage IC high grade mixed mucinous and endometrioid type with clear cell carcinoma; (c) stage IA high-grade serous carcinoma; and (d) stage IIB high grade serous and endometrioid carcinoma. Cases a and b experienced a sharp increase in CA125 values, whereas cases c and d experienced a gradual rise of CA125 within the normal range (< 35U/mL) indicated by the dashed line. (From Ref. 21 with permission.)

(P = 0.021; Figure 1.4) (27). With additional follow-up to 16.3 years, however, no significant difference was shown in deaths due to tubal or ovarian cancer across the control, TVS and multimodality groups (28). While mortality was not decreased, screening with CA125 followed by TVS did increase the fraction of early stage (I–II) cases by 13% and reduced late stage (III–IV) disease by 11% compared with the unscreened population. Multimodality screening had a sensitivity of 52% for detecting ovarian cancer and was associated with increased use of primary surgery (P < 0.0001), increased zero residual disease after cytoreduction (P < 0.0001) and increased use of both surgery and chemotherapy (P = 0.0032) (29). After 18 years, there was a 6.9% improvement in survival in the multimodal group (P = 0.042) without an overall impact on mortality. Remarkably, only 15% of patients with screen-detected stage IA/B

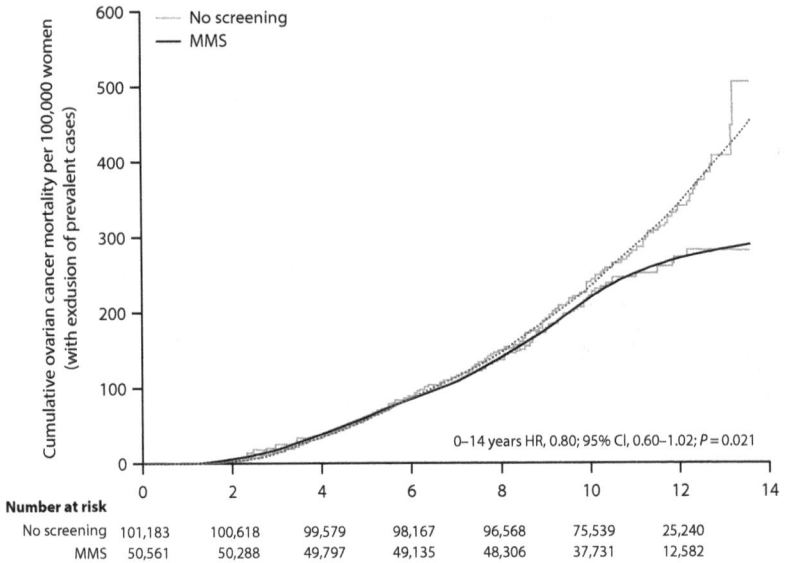

FIGURE 1.4 Cumulative ovarian cancer deaths. In the UKCTOCS trial reported in 2016. HR, hazard ratio; Multimodality Screening (black) vs control (gray). (From Ref. 21 with permission.)

ovarian cancers received optimal combination chemotherapy with platinum and a taxane. While data for stage IC and II cancers are not available, only 60% of patients with stage IC to IV disease received combination chemotherapy. Currently, in the United States, NCCN (National Comprehensive Cancer Network) guidelines recommend combination chemotherapy for all stages of invasive ovarian cancer both high grade and non-high grade. Inadequate treatment would extend survival in incident cases, but not reduce mortality in the long term, consistent with the transient decrease in apparent mortality observed in the UKCTOCs (Figure 1.4) that did not persist with longer follow-up. The two-stage strategy did achieve adequate specificity, as indicated by a 22% PPV, with just over 4 operations required to detect each case of ovarian cancer.

The NROSS trial evaluated the same multimodal screening strategy in a single arm study conducted in the United States over the last 21 years in parallel with the UKCTOCS (30, 31). Some 7,856 healthy postmenopausal women at average risk for ovarian cancer were screened annually for a total of 50,596 woman-years using CA125 analyzed with the ROCA followed by TVS in 2% of subjects annually. Screening prompted 34 operations to detect 17 ovarian cancers – 15 invasive high grade and 2 borderline – with 12 (70%) in stage I or II (31). CA125 and the ROCA missed 6 ovarian cancers, so the sensitivity of the screen for detecting ovarian and borderline cancer was 74% (17/23). Interestingly, 7 endometrial cancers were also detected with 6 in stage I. The positive predictive value (PPV) of this strategy was 50% (17/34) for ovarian cancer and 74% (25/34) for any cancer, far exceeding the study endpoint of a 10% PPV. Remarkably, 70% of screen-detected ovarian cancers and borderline tumors (12/17) were detected in early stage (I–II). Furthermore, of the 19 invasive epithelial ovarian cancers diagnosed by screening [15] or clinically [4], 11 of 19 (58%) were identified in early stage. Only 2 operations were required to detect each case of ovarian cancer, consistent with the 3–4 operations required in the UKCTOCS, indicating that CA125 used in this way is indeed adequately specific for screening (31).

1.3.4 Stage Shift and Mortality

In the multimodal screening (MMS) arm of the UKCTOCS trial, early stage (I–II) disease increased from 24% in controls to 38% with significantly rising CA125 followed by TVS, an absolute difference of only 14% (27). Using the same control, a stage shift of 34% was observed in the NROSS trial where early stage (I–II) disease increased from 24% to 58%. In screening trials, a large relative late-stage reduction has been linked to a significant reduction in mortality. Compared to the UKCTOCS control arm at 76%, NROSS reduced the proportion of cases in late stage (III–IV) disease to 42%, a reduction of 34%. Compared to 60.5% distant disease in US SEER populations, NROSS reduced distant disease to 30.5%, a reduction of 30%. By contrast, the UKCTOCS MMS arm reported a reduction in the proportion of late-stage disease by only 14%.

While the stage shift in the UKCTOCS was statistically significant, the 14% magnitude reduction in late-stage disease may not have been sufficient to reduce mortality (32). In screening for breast and lung cancer, the magnitude of stage shift has been critical for mortality reduction (33). Across multiple randomized trials of mammography to detect early stage breast cancer, trials that achieved a reduction in the incidence of late stage disease of 20% or greater had a statistically significant mortality reduction, whereas those with less than a 20% stage shift did not (34).

The reason for a greater stage shift observed in the smaller NROSS trial is not clear (32). Differences could simply reflect statistical variation, but other factors could have affected results. Accuracy of TVS imaging might have affected the overall outcome of the two trials. In a retrospective review of TVS in the UKCTOCS, fallopian tubes and ovaries could be identified in only 50% of 1000 archived cases (35). In studies of quality control conducted at the University of Kentucky, fallopian tubes and ovaries were visualized in more than 75% of cases (36). Methods for processing blood for the CA125 assay differed between the two studies. In the NROSS, blood for CA125 was drawn in glass tubes without gel and serum was separated and frozen at -80°C on the same day. In the UKCTOCS, blood was drawn in gel separation tubes, shipped to the central lab in London at ambient temperature and separated and frozen within a limit of 56 hours from subject's blood draw to sample processing. As the ROCA can detect subtle changes in CA125, degradation of CA125 protein could affect the results, particularly with low levels of CA125. A modest systematic reduction in CA125 levels in the UKCTOCS could have decreased the ability to detect early-stage disease. In addition, particular care was taken in the NROSS to follow elevated CA125 with repeated TVS to minimize time to surgery. The median time from last CA125 value to surgery was 32 days (31).

1.3.5 Cost Effectiveness

The cost effectiveness of two-stage screening strategies has been evaluated with several models for women at average risk (37–39). Using models that reduce mortality by 13–15%, estimates have ranged from $88,993 to $106,187 per quality adjusted life year. Cost effectiveness improved when populations at higher risk were considered (37).

1.4 SCREENING WOMEN AT HIGH RISK

The lifetime risk of developing ovarian cancer incidence in the general population is approximately 1.3%, but this risk increases dramatically in women with germ-line mutations of BRCA1 (39–46%) or BRCA2 (10–28%) (40, 41). Approximately 15–24% of patients with high grade serous carcinomas carry mutant BRCA1 or BRCA2 genes in their germline and a small additional fraction exhibit somatic BRCA mutations (41). Both Li-Fraumeni syndrome, caused by germ line mutation of TP53, and Lynch syndrome, resulting from germ line mutations in DNA, mismatch repair genes (*MLH1, MSH2, MSH6, MLH3* and *PMS2*) which can also predispose to epithelial ovarian cancer. Risk-reducing bilateral salpingo-oophorectomy can substantially reduce the risk of ovarian cancer in patients affected by these hereditary cancer syndromes (42), but is often delayed until childbearing is completed. During this interval, CA125 and TVS may be performed semi-annually starting at age 30–35, although guidelines provided by several organizations do not recommend their use in the absence of data to demonstrate that such surveillance reduces mortality (41).

When screening was performed annually with the ROCA followed by TVS in 3,563 asymptomatic women with high risk (at > 10% risk) of developing ovarian cancer in phase I of the UK Familial Ovarian Cancer Screening Study (UKFOCSS), the sensitivity for detecting ovarian cancer was 81%, but only 31% (4/13) were in stage I or II (43). When screening was performed every 4 months with the ROCA followed by TVS in 4,348 women at > 10% risk in phase 2 of the UKFOCSS, 38% (5/13) of screen-detected cancers were in stage I or II (44). Six women were diagnosed with ovarian cancer having elected to have risk-reducing surgery (RRS) while on this study and 5 of 6 were in stage I. If these cases were included, 53% (10/19) were in stage I or II. After screening ended, participants continued to be followed. While 37% (7/19) of women who were diagnosed with ovarian cancer within one year after screening ended were in late stage (stage IIIb–IV), 94% (17/18) were in late stage when diagnosed at a later interval, indicating a substantial stage shift was associated with screening.

A similar strategy was used in two US trials that screened 3,692 women at elevated risk with the ROCA and TVS every 3 months (45). Overall, 19 cases of ovarian cancer were detected. Four were prevalent, 6 incident and 9 detected at RRS. Among the incident cases, 3 of 6 (50%) were in early stage (I–II) and 6 of 9 cancers (67%) found at RRS were in stage I. Early-stage patients experienced progression free survival of 6 years. An increase in early-stage disease is encouraging but does not prove a reduction in mortality. With the very high risk of ovarian cancer in this population, randomized screening trials where patients are randomized to no screening are unlikely to be acceptable. With mortality as the endpoint, large cohorts of high-risk women who wish to postpone RRS and willing to risk randomization to no screening would need to be identified, which is also very unlikely. Hence it is not likely that answers to the question of whether screening of high-risk women reduces ovarian cancer mortality will ever be obtained.

1.5 IMPROVING THE INITIAL STAGE OF SCREENING

As only 80% of ovarian cancers express CA125 at a tissue level and blood levels of CA125 are increased in only 50–70% of early stage (I–II) cases, additional biomarkers might detect cases missed by CA125, improving sensitivity of the initial stage of screening. Biomarkers might also be sought with low levels in healthy women and increased shedding from small ovarian cancers.

A model developed by Brown and Palmer estimated high grade serous cancers progressed to an advanced stage (III–IV) when their diameter reached approximately 3 cm (43). If their model accurately reflects ovarian cancer biology, to achieve a sensitivity of 50%, a screening strategy would need to detect cancers of 1.3 cm in diameter and a 50% reduction in mortality would require detecting 0.5 cm cancers. Hori and Gambhir estimated that a tumor size of 2.5 cm would be required to elevate CA125 in blood above the standard cutoff (46). Based on recent pathology reports in the NROSS trial, screen-detected cancers averaged 10.2 cm in stage I and 9.4 cm in stage II with the smallest stage I lesion measuring 4 cm in largest diameter, consistent with estimates from Hori & Gambhir.

1.5.1 Development of a Multi-biomarker Panel

Over the last two decades, the authors have evaluated more than 130 biomarkers to identify those that complement CA125 in detecting early-stage ovarian cancer (21). From our own studies and from the literature, 35 biomarkers have been identified that complement CA125 that might improve the sensitivity of the initial step in screening (21, 47–50).

1.5.1.1 Protein antigens

CA-125 is a heavily glycosylated high molecular weight (1–5 million Daltons) mucin protein (MUC16) whose levels can be elevated in the blood by several conditions including ovarian cancer (51). CA125 is cleaved and shed from the cell surface by proteolysis. Blood levels of CA125 correlate with levels in cancer tissue and with tumor burden (17, 18).

CA125 can be elevated in 50–60 % of early stage (I–II) ovarian cancers and in up to 90% of late-stage (III–IV) disease where inflamed normal mesothelial cells can elevate CA125 levels. HE4 is a 25 kD secreted protein found to be elevated in sera from 73% of all stages ovarian cancers at 89% specificity in a meta-analysis (52). Although HE4 is slightly less sensitive than CA125, as it detects only 40–50% of early stage (I–II) ovarian cancers, but has better specificity for distinguishing malignant from benign pelvic masses (53, 54). HE4 is twice as sensitive as CA125 for detecting endometrial cancer with elevated HE4 levels in 36% of all stages and 17% of stage I endometrial cancers. CA125 levels are more affected than HE4 by menstrual cycle, smoking, oral contraceptive use and age (55). While both CA125 and HE4 levels are elevated in serous and endometrioid ovarian cancers (55), they tend to be lower in the mucinous subtype, whereas CA72.4 is highly elevated in mucinous ovarian cancers (55). For early-stage ovarian cancer detection, previous studies have examined CA125 and HE4 in combination with other biomarkers including CA72.4 (56), CA72.4 and CA15-3 (57), CEA and V-CAM1 (58), glycodelin (59), E-cadherin and IL-6 (59) or transthyretin (61).

Two different algorithms, the Risk of Malignancy Algorithm (ROMA) (60) and OVA1 (OVERA) (18, 63) were approved by the FDA to distinguish ovarian cancers from benign pelvic masses, informing referral of patients to gynecologic oncologists with appropriate expertise. ROMA is an algorithm which combines CA125 and HE4 with menopausal status, providing 94% sensitivity for distinguishing malignant from benign lesions at 75% specificity with a high negative predictive value of 99%. OVERA is a multivariate index calculated by combining data from imaging, menopausal status and CA125 and HE4 with three other biomarkers (transferrin, apolipoprotein A1 and follicle-stimulating hormone) providing 93% sensitivity at 69% specificity with a negative predictive value (NPV) of 99% (18, 63). One report suggests that OVERA might detect more cancers than ROMA (18).

There are other protein antigens associated with ovarian cancer. Using immuno-peroxidase staining of tissue arrays, we assessed expression of 10 potential serum tumor markers developed by other groups in 65 epithelial ovarian cancers with little or no CA125 expression and in ovarian cystadenomas, tumors of low malignant potential, normal ovaries and 16 other normal tissues (64). In ovarian cancers that lacked CA125, all specimens (100%) expressed human kallikrein 10 (HK10), human kallikrein 6 (HK6), osteopontin (OPN) and claudin 3. A smaller fraction of CA125-deficient ovarian cancers expressed DF3, endothelial growth factor (VEGF), MUC1, mesothelin (SMRP), HE4 and CA19-9. When reactivity with normal tissues was considered, mesothelin and HE4 showed the greatest specificity. Osteopontin, a glycophosphoprotein, is secreted into body fluids by normal osteoblasts, arterial smooth muscle cells, epithelial cells, activated T cells and macrophages, but can also be overexpressed by multiple cancers including ovarian cancer and could be used as clinical biomarker (61–64, 66). OPN is elevated in 20–50% of early-stage and 20–46% late-stage ovarian cancers and detects 14–38% of patients missed by CA125 (59). HK6 and HK10 were reported as potential prognostic biomarkers in ovarian cancer (65, 66). HK6 and HK10 are secreted serine proteases which are highly expressed in ovarian tissue (67) and are elevated in sera from 50% of late-stage cases (67). HK6 detected 9% and HK10 detected 14% of early-stage ovarian cancers, while HK6 and HK10 together detected only 6% of CA125-negative early-stage cases.

The increased sensitivity achieved with combined biomarker panels leads to a decrease in specificity. However, machine learning algorithms and statistical analysis, including neural networks and multivariate mixture models, reflecting the mixture of tumor biomarkers, can increase sensitivity with panels of biomarkers, while maintaining a fixed target specificity. Combining biomarker panel, CA125, CA15-3, CA72-4 and M-CSF were assayed in sera from patients with stage I ovarian cancer and from healthy individuals, sensitivity was increased from 48% with CA125 alone to 72% with artificial neural network analysis and to 75% with a multivariate mixture model of the panel, while maintaining specificity at 98% (68, 69).

In a collaborative project with EDRN investigators, a panel of 952 sera were assembled where CA125 detected 72% of early stage (I–II) ovarian cancers at 98% specificity whereas a combination of CA125, HE4, HE4 antigen-autoantibody complexes and OPN detected 91% of early-stage cases at 93% specificity (70). Using Random Forest analysis to achieve 98% specificity, the four-biomarker panel significantly (p = 0.003) improved sensitivity over CA125 by 13% (70). Consequently, these four biomarkers were chosen for second generation algorithm development.

Based on this analysis, a new longitudinal ROCA2 algorithm has been developed that combines values for the four-biomarker panel over time using hierarchical change-point and multivariate mixture models for the longitudinal values from the cases and a hierarchical longitudinal baseline model for the controls (women not diagnosed with ovarian cancer during screening and follow-up). Inference for the parameters in the model was obtained through Markov chain Monte-Carlo (MCMC) sampling. For any new sequence over time of the four biomarkers, the Bayes factor was calculated to assess the likelihood that any one or more of the four markers had a change-point. The Bayes factor then updates the prior odds based on age to estimate the posterior odds which are then straightforwardly transformed to the estimate of risk of having ovarian cancer. Screening decisions such as referral to TVS are then made based on the latest value of the risk. This algorithm will be tested in the NROSS2 trial funded by the NCI Early Detection Research Network.

1.5.1.2 Autoantibodies and antigen-autoantibody complexes

Autoantibodies against ovarian cancer associated proteins could, in principle, be stimulated by very small volumes of cancer in the ovary or fallopian tube, providing greater sensitivity and lead time compared to protein biomarkers (71). Some 96% of high-grade serous cancers exhibit TP53 mutations and a majority of these mutations result in decreased degradation and consequent overexpression of TP53 protein. Autoantibodies can be produced against over-expressed TP53 proteins. We found that autoantibodies against TP53 were elevated in 20–28% of > 150 ovarian cancer cases from the UKCTOCS, MD Anderson and Australia (62). In UKCTOCS specimens, anti-TP53 autoantibodies were elevated 8 months before elevation of CA125 and 22 months prior to clinical diagnosis when CA125 was not elevated (72).

Autoantibodies against TP53, prostaglandin F receptor and protein tyrosine phosphatase receptor type A 1 were the most prevalent in a screen of 5,177 autoantigens (73). A sensitivity of 23% for all stages could be achieved at 98% specificity, when levels of 2 of the 3 autoantibodies were elevated. A panel of autoantibodies against TP53, TRIM-21, NY-ESO-1 (CTAG-1A) and PAX-8 together showed a sensitivity of 46–56% at a specificity of 98% for all stages of ovarian cancer (74).

When 18 different autoantibodies were assayed in 952 sera assembled by EDRN investigators, anti-TP53, anti–CTAG1 and anti–IL-8 detected 22% of early stage (I–II) cases and 3% of those missed by CA125 (70). Anna Lokshin has reported that anti–CTAG1 and anti–IL-8 autoantibodies can be elevated 18 months prior to diagnosis (personal communication).

Autoantibodies against HE4 and HE4 antigen-autoantibody complexes have been measured in sera from patients with early stage (I–II) ovarian cancers (75). While free autoantibodies were observed in less than 6% of cases, HE4 antigen-autoantibody complexes were found in 39% of early-stage cases at 98% specificity (75). With the EDRN Discovery Panel, HE4 antigen-autoantibody complexes detected 19% of early-stage cases and 33% of CA125-negative cases. Use of CA125 and HE4 antigen-autoantibody complexes in combination increase the fraction of cases detected from 63% with CA125 alone to 81% with both biomarkers (75).

1.5.1.3 Non-coding RNA

MicroRNAs are small non-coding RNAs of 20–25 nucleotides in length that regulate protein expression. Serum levels of circulating miRNAs are promising candidates for early detection of ovarian cancer (76). Changes in multiple miRNA levels in ovarian cancer cells or tissue have been correlated with proliferation, migration, invasion, apoptosis and chemosensitivity (77). miRNAs have also been detected in exosomal vesicles separated from sera or obtained from cultured ovarian cancer cells (78). From a review of the literature, at least 15 miRNAs are upregulated and 9 are downregulated in serum or plasma from ovarian cancer patients (77). Neural network analysis of 9 miRNAs has been used to distinguish malignant from benign pelvic masses, achieving a PPV of 91.3% and a NPV of 78.6% and 0.90 AUC (76). A distinct panel of 10 miRNAs was evaluated in 4,046 multi-cancer and control serum samples, including 428 cases of ovarian tumor. A model was developed that distinguished ovarian cancer cases from healthy control with 99% sensitivity and 100% specificity but failed to distinguish controls from borderline cancer or benign pelvic masses (79). These data require confirmation. To date, miRNAs individually or as panels have not shown complementarity with CA125 (80).

1.5.1.4 DNA

Cell-free DNA (cfDNA) is extracellular DNA (double-stranded or mitochondrial) that can be derived from normal or malignant cells often as a result of apoptosis and necrosis. Circulating tumor DNA (ctDNA), derived specifically from tumor cells, can be present in plasma and can function as a clinical biomarker (81). ctDNA in blood and cervical secretions can be detected in 55% of early-stage ovarian cancers and complements CA125 for further improvement in early detection (82). In general, the volume of tumors must be > 1 cm in diameter to elevate ctDNA in blood. Development of a repetitive element aneuploidy sequencing system (RealSeq) to detect aneuploidy in ctDNA from as little as 3 pg of DNA in liquid biopsies promises to improve sensitivity for detecting early-stage high grade ovarian cancers with copy number abnormalities (83).

Despite the potential utility of ctDNA for early detection, its short half-life (30 min to 2hrs) and large volume of plasma required for ctDNA analysis have been major challenges for retrospective analysis from serum banks. Somatic mutations in clonal hematopoietic stem cells of indeterminate potential (CHIP) further complicate detection of early-stage cancers based on DNA mutations.

1.5.1.5 DNA methylation

When the methylation status of seven genes – *APC, RASSF1A, CHDH1, RUNX3, TFP12, SRP5 and OPCML* – was compared in sera from early-stage ovarian cancer cases and from healthy individuals, the panel achieved 85% sensitivity at 91% specificity for early stage disease, compared to 56% sensitivity and 64% specificity for CA125 alone (84). Another panel of three genes was measured in cell-free DNA from the control arm of the UKCTOCS trial where 57.9% of women who developed ovarian cancer within 2 years were detected at a specificity of 88.1% (85). The sensitivity of these assays has not been reported at the 98% specificity required for cost-effective two-stage screening.

1.5.1.6 Metabolites

Metabolites have also been evaluated as biomarkers for early detection (86, 87). The majority of metabolites (95%) have been assayed with mass spectrometry (78). Drs. Johannes Fahrmann and Samir Hanash demonstrated that a plasma polyamine signature provided a promising biomarker and complemented CA125 for detecting early-stage ovarian cancer. Using mass spectrometry profiling, a polyamine signature consisting of diacetylspermine (DAS) + N-(3-acetamidopropyl) pyrrolidin-2-one (N3A) in combination with CA125 improved sensitivity at > 99% specificity to 74% compared to 62% with CA125 alone (P = 0.019), capturing 30% of cases that were missed with CA125 (93). They established a deep learning model that combined ROMA (CA125, HE4 and menopausal status) with a panel of 7 circulating polyamine metabolites and that showed significant improvement (P < 0.001) with an increase of PPV by 16% (0.68 vs. 0.52; P < 0.001) and specificity by 11% compared with ROMA alone for distinguishing early stage ovarian cancer from benign pelvic masses (94).

1.6 MULTI-CANCER SCREENING

Screening for multiple cancers (ovary, liver, stomach, pancreas and esophagus) is being tested in populations at conventional risk through assessment of the levels of cell-free DNA and circulating protein (88). CancerSEEK combined DNA sequencing to identify cancer relevant mutations and protein biomarkers (CA125) to detect ovarian cancer with 98% sensitivity at 99% specificity among a group of 1,005 patients with different types of cancer. However, 76% of patients detected were in stage III with long-term survival < 30%. In this setting, CA125 alone exhibits > 90% sensitivity at 97% specificity. In the subsequent DETECT-A study of 10,006 apparently healthy women, this approach to multi-cancer screening detected 50 cancers. Testing for ctDNA mutations and protein biomarkers identified 26 cancers with 15 cases confirmed by PET-CT; 24 cases were detected by conventional methods (89). With combined PET-CT and blood testing, sensitivity increased from 98.9% to 99.6%, whereas PPV was increased from 19.4% to 28.3%. Among the 26 cancers detected, 6 were ovarian (23%) but only one was in early stage (17%). To assure specificity, the CA125 threshold was set high at 577 U/mL, 16 times higher than usual threshold of CA125 (35U/ml), which would have missed all 17 early-stage cancers found in the NROSS (31). While multi-cancer screening is an attractive concept, predictive performance of CancerSEEK for detection of early stage is limited and needs to be improved.

1.7 IMPROVING THE SECOND STAGE OF SCREENING WITH BETTER IMAGING

Precise imaging of ovarian cancer has been a challenge and has become a major hurdle for improving detection of early-stage ovarian cancer (20). A fraction of high grade serous ovarian cancers arises from epithelial cells on the fallopian tubes, which cannot be easily imaged. The specificity and sensitivity of TVS is limited. Review of TVS in the UKCTOCS indicated that fallopian tubes and ovaries could only be identified in 50% of 1,000 archived cases (35). Studies from the University of Kentucky suggest that more than 75% of fallopian tubes and images can be imaged (36), Doppler flow (90) or use of microbubbles (91) that characterize blood flow within the tumor improve specificity but not sensitivity.

Standardization of TVS using an International Ovarian Tumor Analysis (IOTA) simplifies interpretations of TVS imaging and provides consistency in defining morphological features of ovarian masses. The sensitivity for the detection of malignant cases amongst patients with pelvic masses with IOTA was 91.7%, the specificity was 84.8% and accuracy was 86.7% (92). In the cross-sectional prospective study with 205 women undergoing surgery, including 183 cancer cases, IOTA showed 92.8% sensitivity and specificity was 92.9%. Of the tumors, 144 were benign and 39 were malignant (93).

Multiple strategies have been developed to improve imaging techniques. Hyperpolarized ^{13}C MRI has shown to be effective in prostate cancers and can be applied to ovarian cancer. Photoacoustic imaging can detect early tumor vascularization, but this technique is limited to a tissue depth of 5 cm with a decline in spatial resolution with increasing depth. Combination of photoacoustic tomography with ultrasound can, however, partially compensate for these limitations (94). Falloposcopy is another way to achieve precise imaging of the fallopian tube and ovary required for surveillance of high-risk women with ovarian cancer. Based on its design and combination with optical coherence tomography, imaging of sub-1 mm diameter package could be achievable and diagnosis could be improved (95).

Superconducting Quantum Interference Detection (SQUID) showed promising sensitivity to detect faint magnetic fields measuring delay in magnetic relaxation of antibody-coated iron oxide nanoparticles (96, 97). To provide a visual probe to detect ovarian cancer, anti-CA125 antibodies were conjugated with ferritin nanospheres. When antibody-conjugated nanospheres bind to ovarian cancer cells, relaxation of the magnetic field is delayed, while unbound nanoparticles fail to give a signal. By measuring this delay in magnetic relaxation (MRx), this technique was able to detect a minimal size of 10^6 ovarian cancer cells (0.1 mm) ex-vivo. Compared with current techniques (CT, MRI and PET-CT), which can only provide images enabling detection of 3-5 mm cancer nodules, SQUID imaging significantly could increase detection by 1–2 orders of magnitude (98).

1.8 CONCLUSIONS

The NROSS and UKCTOCS with two-stage screening using CA125 followed by TVS demonstrated adequate specificity and PPV for early detection of ovarian cancer. Failure of the UKCTOCS trial to achieve a reduction in mortality relates to limited sensitivity, a modest stage shift and inadequate chemotherapy by current standards. Higher sensitivity for early-stage disease, a large reduction in late-stage cases and a large and increased PPV in the NROSS are encouraging. It appears that the ROCA can be improved by the addition of other biomarkers including protein antigens and antigen-autoantibody. Recent development of the ROCA2 algorithm and elevation of autoantibodies will be evaluated in the next phase of screening clinical trials. Autoantibodies may provide lead time in a fraction of women screened. If sufficient specificity and sensitivity for early-stage disease can be achieved with improved lead time, a randomized trial powered to observe a mortality advantage should be considered. Meanwhile, precise imaging techniques and machine learning–based statistical models leveraging the power of each subject serving as her/his own control will be also required to advance screening strategy.

ACKNOWLEDGEMENTS

This work was supported by funds from the NCI Early Detection Research Network (5 U01 CA200462 (RC Bast), 5 U01 CA152990 and U2C 271871 (SJ Skates)), the MD Anderson Ovarian SPOREs (P50 CA83639 (RC Bast) and P50CA217685 (RC Bast)), R01 CA247220 (A Lokshin and RC Bast MPIs), National Cancer Institute, Department of Health and Human Services; the Cancer Prevention Research Institute of Texas (RP160145; RC Bast); Golfer's Against Cancer; the Tracey Joe Wilson Foundation; National Foundation for Cancer Research; UT MD Anderson Women's Moon Shot; and generous donations from the Ann and Henry Zarrow Foundation, the Mossy Foundation, the Roberson Endowment, the Walmart Foundation, Stuart and Gaye Lynn Zarrow, Barry and Karen Elson, Arthur and Sandra Williams and from the Concord (MA) Detect Ovarian Cancer Early Fund.

REFERENCES

1. Siegel RL, Miller KD, Wagle NS, Jemal A. Cancer statistics, 2023. *CA Cancer J Clin* 2023;**73**(1):17–48.
2. Sung H, Ferlay J, Siegel RL, *et al.* Global Cancer Statistics 2020: GLOBOCAN Estimates of Incidence and Mortality Worldwide for 36 Cancers in 185 Countries. *CA Cancer J Clin* 2021;**71**(3):209–49.

3. Sep2023. *Stages of Ovarian Cancer.* https://ocrahope.org/get-the-facts/staging. Accessed 2023 Sep2023.
4. Havrilesky LJ, Sanders GD, Kulasingam S, *et al.* Development of an ovarian cancer screening decision model that incorporates disease heterogeneity: implications for potential mortality reduction. *Cancer* 2011;**117**(3):545–53.
5. Jacobs I, Bast RC, Jr. The CA 125 tumour-associated antigen: a review of the literature. *Hum Reprod* 1989;**4**(1):1–12.
6. Bast RC, Jr., Zbar B, Borsos T, Rapp HJ. BCG and cancer (first of two parts). *N Engl J Med* **290**(25):1413–20, 6/1974.
7. Bast RC, Jr., Zbar B, Borsos T, Rapp HJ. BCG and cancer (second of two parts). *N Engl J Med* **290**(26):1458–69, 6/1974.
8. Zbar B, Bernstein ID, Bartlett, GL, et al. Immunotherapy of Cancer: Regression of Intradermal Tumors and Prevention of Growth of Lymph Node Metastases After Intralesional Injection of Living *Mycobacterium bovis. J Natl Cancer Inst* 1972 **49**:119–30, doi: 10.1093/jnci/49.1.119
9. Knapp RC, Berkowitz RS. Corynebacterium parvum as an immunotherapeutic agent in an ovarian cancer model. *Am J Obstet Gynecol* 1977; **128**(7):782–6; doi: 10.1016/0002-9378(77)90721-9
10. Bast RC, Knapp RC, Mitchell AK, Thurston JG, et al. Immunotherapy of a murine ovarian carcinoma with Corynebacterium parvum and specific heteroantiserum. I. Activation of peritoneal cells to mediate antibody-dependent cytotoxicity. *J Immunol* **123**(5):1945–51, November 1979.
11. Bast RC, Berek JS, Obrist R, Griffiths CT, et al. Intraperitoneal immunotherapy of human ovarian carcinoma with Corynebacterium parvum. *Cancer Res* **43**(3):1395–1401, March 1983.
12. Bast RC, Jr., Feeney M, Lazarus H, et al. Reactivity of a monoclonal antibody with human ovarian carcinoma. *J Clin Invest* 1981;**68**(5):1331–7.
13. Yin BW, Lloyd KO. Molecular cloning of the CA125 ovarian cancer antigen: identification as a new mucin, MUC16. *J Biol Chem* 2001; **276**(29):27371–5. doi: 10.1074/jbc.M103554200
14. Fendrick JL, Staley K, Gee MK, Mc Dougald SR, Quirk JG Jr, O'Brien TJ. Characterization of CA 125 synthesized by the human epithelial amnion WISH cell line. *Tumour Biol* 1993;**14**(5):310–8. doi: 10.1159/000217844
15. Bast RC, Jr., Klug TL, St John E, *et al.* A radioimmunoassay using a monoclonal antibody to monitor the course of epithelial ovarian cancer. *N Engl J Med* 1983;**309**(15):883–7.
16. Rustin JG, van der Burg, Griffin CL, Guthrie D et al. Early versus delayed treatment of relapsed ovarian cancer (MRC OVO5/EORTC 55955): a randomised trial. *Lancet* 2010;**376**(9747):1155–63. doi: 10.1016/S0140-6736(10)61268-8
17. Moore RG, Jabre-Raughley M, Brown AK, Robison KM, et al. Comparison of a novel multiple marker assay vs the Risk of Malignancy Index for the prediction of epithelial ovarian cancer in patients with a pelvic mass. *Am J Obstet Gynecol* 2010; **203**(3):228 e1–6. doi: 10.1016/j.ajog.2010.03.043
18. Coleman RL, Herzog TJ, Chan DW, Munroe DG, et al. Validation of a second-generation multivariate index assay for malignancy risk of adnexal masses. *Gynecologie* 2016; **215**(1):82.e1–82.e11. doi: 10.1016/j.ajog.2016.03.003

19. van Nagell JR, Jr., Burgess BT, Miller RW, *et al.* Survival of Women With Type I and II Epithelial Ovarian Cancer Detected by Ultrasound Screening. *Obstet Gynecol* 2018;**132**(5):1091 100.

20. Mathieu KB, Bedi DG, Thrower SL, et al. Screening for ovarian cancer: imaging challenges and opportunities for improvement. *Ultrasound Obstet Gynecol* 2018;**51**(3):293–303.

21. Bast RC, Jr., Lu Z, Han CY, *et al.* Biomarkers and Strategies for Early Detection of Ovarian Cancer. *Cancer Epidemiol Biomarkers Prev* 2020;**29**(12):2504–12.

22. Buys SS, Partridge E, Greene MH, *et al.* Ovarian cancer screening in the Prostate, Lung, Colorectal and Ovarian (PLCO) cancer screening trial: findings from the initial screen of a randomized trial. *Am J Obstet Gynecol* 2005;**193**(5): 1630–9.

23. Kobayashi H, Yamada Y, Sado T, *et al.* A randomized study of screening for ovarian cancer: a multicenter study in Japan. *Int J Gynecol Cancer* 2008; **18**(3):414–20.

24. Skates SJ, Xu FJ, Yu YH, *et al.* Toward an optimal algorithm for ovarian cancer screening with longitudinal tumor markers. *Cancer* 1995;**76**(10 Suppl):2004–10.

25. Skates SJ, Menon U, MacDonald N, *et al.* Calculation of the risk of ovarian cancer from serial CA-125 values for preclinical detection in postmenopausal women. *J Clin Oncol* 2003;**21**(10 Suppl):206s–10s.

26. Menon U, Ryan A, Kalsi J, et al. Risk Algorithm Using Serial Biomarker Measurements Doubles the Number of Screen-Detected Cancers Compared With a Single-Threshold Rule in the United Kingdom Collaborative Trial of Ovarian Cancer Screening. *J Clin Oncol* 2015;**33**(18):2062–71.

27. Jacobs IJ, Menon U, Ryan A, et al. Ovarian cancer screening and mortality in the UK Collaborative Trial of Ovarian Cancer Screening (UKCTOCS): a randomised controlled trial. *Lancet* 2016;**387**(10022):945–56..

28. Menon U, Gentry-Maharaj A, Burnell M, et al. Ovarian cancer population screening and mortality after long-term follow-up in the UK Collaborative Trial of Ovarian Cancer Screening (UKCTOCS): a randomised controlled trial. *Lancet* 2021;**397**(10290):2182–93.

29. Menon U, Gentry-Maharaj A, Burnell M, et al. Tumour stage, treatment and survival of women with high-grade serous tubo-ovarian cancer in UKCTOCS: an exploratory analysis of a randomized controlled trial. *Lancet Oncol* 2023; **24**:1018–28.

30. Lu KH, Skates S, Hernandez MA, *et al.* A 2-stage ovarian cancer screening strategy using the Risk of Ovarian Cancer Algorithm (ROCA) identifies early-stage incident cancers and demonstrates high positive predictive value. *Cancer* 2013;**119**(19):3454–61.

31. Han CY, Lu KH, Corrigan G,et al. The Normal Risk Ovarian Screening Study (NROSS): 21-year update. *J Clin Oncol*, 2024 Jan 9: JCO2300141. doi: 10.1200/JCO.23.00141

32. Bast RC, Han CY, Lu Z, Lu KH. Next steps in the early detection of ovarian cancer. *Commun Med* 2021;**1**.

33. Lee S, Zelen M. A stochastic model for predicting the mortality of breast cancer. *J Natl Cancer Inst Monogr* 2006;(36):79–86.

34. Tabar L, Yen AM, Wu WY, *et al*. Insights from the breast cancer screening trials: how screening affects the natural history of breast cancer and implications for evaluating service screening programs. *Breast J* 2015;**21**(1):13–20.
35. Stott W, Campbell S, Franchini A, *et al*. Sonographers' self-reported visualization of normal postmenopausal ovaries on transvaginal ultrasound is not reliable: results of expert review of archived images from UKCTOCS. *Ultrasound Obstet Gynecol* 2018;**51**(3):401–8.
36. Lefringhouse JR, Neward E, Ueland FR, *et al*. Probability of fallopian tube and ovarian detection with transvaginal ultrasonography in normal women. *Womens Health (London)* 2016;**12**(3):303–11.
37. Drescher CW, Hawley S, Thorpe JD, *et al*. Impact of 6 test performance and cost on mortality reduction and cost-effectiveness of multimodal ovarian cancer screening. *Cancer Prev Res* 2012;**5**(8):1015–24.
38. Sroczynski G, Gogollari A, Kuehne F, *et al*. A Systematic Review on Cost-effectiveness Studies Evaluating Ovarian Cancer Early Detection and Prevention Strategies. *Cancer Prev Res* 2020;**13**(5):429–42.
39. Moss HA, Berchuck A, Neely ML, et al. Estimating Cost-effectiveness of a 8 Ovarian Cancer Screening Program in the United States: Secondary Analysis of the UK Collaborative Trial of Ovarian Cancer Screening (UKCTOCS). *JAMA Oncol* 2018;**4**(2):190–5.
40. Torre LA, Trabert B, DeSantis CE, *et al*. Ovarian cancer statistics, 2018. *CA Cancer J Clin* 2018;**68**(4):284–96.
41. Lewis KE, Lu KH, Klimczak AM, Mok SC. Recommendations and Choices for BRCA Mutation Carriers at Risk for Ovarian Cancer: A Complicated Decision. *Cancers (Basel)* 2018;**10**(2).
42. Neff RT, Senter L, Salani R. BRCA mutation in ovarian cancer: testing, implications and treatment considerations. *Ther Adv Med Oncol* 2017;**9**(8):519–31.
43. Brown PO, Palmer C. The preclinical natural history of serous ovarian cancer: defining the target for early detection. *PLoS Med* 2009;**6**:e1000114.
44. Rosenthal AN, Fraser LSM, Philpott S, *et al*. Evidence of Stage Shift in Women Diagnosed With Ovarian Cancer During Phase II of the United Kingdom Familial Ovarian Cancer Screening Study. *J Clin Oncol* 2017;**35**(13):1411–20.
45. Skates SJ, Greene MH, Buys SS, *et al*. Early Detection of Ovarian Cancer using the Risk of Ovarian Cancer Algorithm with Frequent CA125 Testing in Women at Increased Familial Risk - Combined Results from Two Screening Trials. *Clin Cancer Res* 2017;**23**(14):3628–37.
46. Hori SS, Gambhir SS. Mathematical model identifies blood biomarker-based early cancer detection strategies and limitations. *Sci Transl Med* 2011;**3**(109):109ra16.
47. Russell MR, Graham C, D'Amato A, *et al*. A combined biomarker panel shows improved sensitivity for the early detection of ovarian cancer allowing the identification of the most aggressive type II tumours. *Br J Cancer* 2017;**117**(5):666–74.
48. Russell MR, Graham C, D'Amato A, *et al*. Diagnosis of epithelial ovarian cancer using a combined protein biomarker panel. *Br J Cancer* 2019;**121**(6):483–9.
49. Whitwell HJ, Worthington J, Blyuss O, *et al*. Improved early detection of ovarian cancer using longitudinal multimarker models. *Br J Cancer* 2020;**122**(6):847–56.
50. Bast RC, Jr. Status of tumor markers in ovarian cancer screening. *J Clin Oncol* 2003;**21**(10 Suppl):200s–5s.

51. Yin BW, Lloyd KO. Molecular cloning of the CA125 ovarian cancer antigen: identification as a new mucin, MUC16. *J Biol Chem* 2001;**276**(29):27371–5.
52. Yang Z, Wei C, Luo Z, Li L. Clinical value of serum human epididymis protein 4 assay in the diagnosis of ovarian cancer: a meta-analysis. *Onco Targets Ther* 2013;**6**:957–66.
53. Moore RG, McMeekin DS, Brown AK, *et al.* A novel multiple marker bioassay utilizing HE4 and CA125 for the prediction of ovarian cancer in patients with a pelvic mass. *Gynecol Oncol* 2009;**112**(1):40–6.
54. Hellstrom I, Raycraft J, Hayden-Ledbetter M, *et al.* The HE4 (WFDC2) protein is a biomarker for ovarian carcinoma. *Cancer Res* 2003;**63**(13):3695–700.
55. Simmons AR, Baggerly K, Bast RC, Jr. The emerging role of HE4 in the evaluation of epithelial ovarian and endometrial carcinomas. *Oncology* 2013;**27**(6):548–56.
56. Simmons AR, Fourkala EO, Gentry-Maharaj A, *et al.* Complementary Longitudinal Serum Biomarkers to CA125 for Early Detection of Ovarian Cancer. *Cancer Prev Res* 2019;**12**(6):391–400.
57. Terry KL, Schock H, Fortner RT, *et al.* A Prospective Evaluation of Early Detection Biomarkers for Ovarian Cancer in the European EPIC Cohort. *Clin Cancer Res* 2016;**22**(18):4664–75.
58. Yurkovetsky Z, Skates S, Lomakin A, et al. Development of a Multimarker assay for early detection of ovarian cancer. *J Clin Oncol* 2010;**28**:2159–66.
59. Blyuss O, Gentry-Maharaj G, Fourkala EO, et al. Serial patterns of ovarian cancer biomarkers in a prediagnosis longitudinal dataset. *Biomed Res Int* 2015;**2015**:681416.
60. Han C, Bellone S, Siegel ER, et al. A novel multiple biomarker panel for the early detection of high-grade serous ovarian carcinoma. *Gynecol Oncol* 2018;**149**:585–91.
61. Zheng X, Chen S, Li L, et al. Evaluation of HE4 and TTR for diagnosis of ovarian cancer: comparison with CA-125. *J Gynecol Obstet Hum Reprod 2018*;**47**:227–30.
62. Moore RG, Miller MC, Disilvestro P, *et al.* Evaluation of the diagnostic accuracy of the risk of ovarian malignancy algorithm in women with a pelvic mass. *Obstet Gynecol* 2011;**118**(2 Pt 1):280–8.
63. Zhang Z, Chan DW. The road from discovery to clinical diagnostics: lessons learned from the first FDA-cleared in vitro diagnostic multivariate index assay of proteomic biomarkers. *Cancer Epidemiol Biomarkers Prev* 2010;**19**(12):2995–9.
64. Rosen DG, Wang L, Atkinson JN, *et al.* Potential markers that complement expression of CA125 in epithelial ovarian cancer. *Gynecol Oncol* 2005;**99**(2):267–77.
65. Ballehaninna UK, Chamberlain RS. Biomarkers for pancreatic cancer: promising new markers and options beyond CA 19-9. *Tumour Biol* 2013;**34**(6):3279–92.
66. Matsuura M, Suzuki T, Saito T. Osteopontin is a new target molecule for ovarian clear cell 2arcinoma therapy. *Cancer Sci* 2010;**101**(8):1828–33.
67. Kim JH, Skates SJ, Uede T, *et al.* Osteopontin as a potential diagnostic biomarker for ovarian cancer. *JAMA* 2002;**287**(13):1671–9.
68. Mor G, Visintin I, Lai Y, *et al.* Serum protein markers for early detection of ovarian cancer. *Proc Natl Acad Sci USA* 2005;**102**(21):7677–82.
69. Guo J, Yang WL, Pak D, *et al.* Osteopontin, Macrophage Migration Inhibitory Factor and Anti-Interleukin-8 Autoantibodies Complement CA125 for Detection of Early Stage Ovarian Cancer. *Cancers* 2019;**11**(5).

70. Luo LY, Katsaros D, Scorilas A, *et al.* The serum concentration of human kallikrein 10 represents a novel biomarker for ovarian cancer diagnosis and prognosis. *Cancer Res* 2003;**63**(4):807–11.
71. Diamandis EP, Yousef GM. Human tissue kallikreins: A family of new cancer biomarkers. *Clin Chem* 2002;**48**(8):1198–205.
72. Diamandis EP, Scorilas A, Fracchioli S, *et al.* Human kallikrein 6 (hK6): A new potential serum biomarker for diagnosis and prognosis of ovarian carcinoma. *J Clin Oncol* 2003;**21**(6):1035–43.
73. Skates SJ, Horick N, Yu Y, *et al.* Preoperative sensitivity and specificity for early-stage ovarian cancer when combining cancer antigen CA-125II, CA 15-3, CA 72-4, and macrophage colony-stimulating factor using mixtures of multivariate normal distributions. *J Clin Oncol* 2004;**22**(20):4059–66.
74. Zhang Z, Yu Y, Xu F, *et al.* Combining multiple serum tumor markers improves detection of stage I epithelial ovarian cancer. *Gynecol Oncol* 2007;**107**(3):526–31.
75. Han CY, Yang W-L, Hawley SJ, et al. Autoantibodies, antigen-autoantibody complexes and antigens that complement CA125 for early detection of ovarian cancer. *British J Cancer* 2024 Jan 9. doi: 10.1038/s41416-023-02560-z
76. Kaaks R, Fortner RT, Husing A, *et al.* Tumor-associated autoantibodies as early detection markers for ovarian cancer? A prospective evaluation. *Int J Cancer* 2018;**143**(3):515–26.
77. Yang WL, Gentry-Maharaj A, Simmons A, *et al.* Elevation of TP53 autoantibody before CA125 in preclinical invasive epithelial ovarian cancer. *Clin Cancer Res* 2017;**23**(19):5912–22.
78. Anderson KS, Cramer DW, Sibani S, *et al.* Autoantibody signature for the serologic detection of ovarian cancer. *J Proteome Res* 2015;**14**(1):578–86.
79. Hurley LC, Levin NK, Chatterjee M, *et al.* Evaluation of paraneoplastic antigens reveals TRIM21 autoantibodies as biomarker for early detection of ovarian cancer in combination with autoantibodies to NY-ESO-1 and TP53. *Cancer Biomark* 2020;**27**(3):407–21.
80. Yang WL, Lu Z, Guo J, *et al.* Human epididymis protein 4 antigen-autoantibody complexes complement cancer antigen 125 for detecting early-stage ovarian cancer. *Cancer* 2020;**126**(4):725–36.
81. Elias KM, Fendler W, Stawiski K, *et al.* Diagnostic potential for a serum miRNA neural network for detection of ovarian cancer. *elife* 2017;**6**: e28932.
82. Staicu CE, Predescu DV, Rusu CM, *et al.* role of micrornas as clinical cancer biomarkers for ovarian cancer: A short overview. *Cells* 2020;**9**(1).
83. Yokoi A, Yoshioka Y, Hirakawa A, *et al.* A combination of circulating miRNAs for the early detection of ovarian cancer. *Oncotarget* 2017;**8**(52):89811–23.
84. Yokoi A, Matsuzaki J, Yamamoto Y, *et al.* Integrated extracellular microRNA profiling for ovarian cancer screening. *Nat Commun* 2018;**9**(1):4319.
85. Elias KM, Guo J, Bast RC, Jr. Early Detection of Ovarian Cancer. *Hematol Oncol Clin North Am* 2018;**32**(6):903–14.
86. Bettegowda C, Sausen M, Leary RJ, *et al.* Detection of circulating tumor DNA in early- and late-stage human malignancies. *Sci Transl Med* 2014;**6**(224):224ra24.
87. Bast RC Jr, Matulonis UA, Sood AK, et al. Critical questions in ovarian cancer research and treatment: report of an American Association for Cancer Research Special Conference. *Cancer* 2019;**125**:1963–72.

88. Douville C, Cohen JD, Ptak J, *et al.* Assessing aneuploidy with repetitive element sequencing. *Proc Natl Acad Sci USA* 2020;**117**(9):4858–63.

89. Zhang Q, Hu G, Yang Q, *et al.* A Multiplex Methylation-Specific PCR Assay for the Detection of early-stage ovarian cancer using cell-free serum DNA. *Gynecol Oncol* 2013;**130**(1):132–9.

90. Widschwendter M, Zikan M, Wahl B, *et al.* The potential of circulating tumor DNA methylation analysis for the early detection and management of ovarian cancer. *Genome Med* 2017;**9**(1):116.

91. Faubert B, Solmonson A, DeBerardinis RJ. Metabolic reprogramming and cancer progression. *Sience* 2020;**368**(6487).

92. Goldsmith P, Fenton H, Morris-Stiff G, et al. Metabonomics: A useful tool for the future surgeon. *J Surg Res* 2010;**160**(1):122–32.

93. Fahrmann JF, Irajizad E, Kobayashi M, *et al.* A MYC-driven plasma polyamine signature for early detection of ovarian cancer. *Cancers* 2021;**13**(4).

94. Irajizad E, Han CY, Celestino J, *et al.* A blood-based metabolite panel for distinguishing ovarian cancer from benign pelvic masses. *Clin Cancer Res* 2022;**28**(21):4669–76.

95. Cohen JD, Li L, Wang Y, *et al.* Detection and localization of surgically resectable cancers with a multi-analyte blood test. *Science* 2018;**359**(6378):926–30.

96. Lennon AM, Buchanan AH, Kinde I, *et al.* Feasibility of blood testing combined with PET-CT to screen for cancer and guide intervention. *Science* 2020; **369**(6499).

97. Medeiros LR, Rosa DD, da Rosa MI, Bozzetti MC. Accuracy of ultrasonography with color Doppler. doi: 10.1111/IGC.0b013e31819c1369

98. Szymanski M, Socha MW, Kowalkowska ME, et al. Differentiating between benign and malignant adnexal lesions with contrast-enhanced transvaginal ultrasonography. *Int J Gynaecol Obstet* 2015;**131**(2):147–51.

99. Garg S, Kaur A, Mohi JK, et al. Evaluation of IOTA simple ultrasound rules to distinguish benign and malignant ovarian tumours. *J Clin Diagn Res* 2017; **11**(8):TC06–TC9.

100. Shetty J, Saradha A, Pandey D, et al. IOTA simple ultrasound rules for triage of adnexal mass: Experience from South India. *J Obstet Gynaecol India* 2019;**69**(4):356–62.

101. Zackrisson S, van de Ven S, Gambhir SS. Light in and sound out: Emerging translational strategies for photoacoustic imaging. *Cancer Res* 2014;**74**(4):979–1004.

102. Keenan M, Tate TH, Kieu K, et al. Design and characterization of a combined OCT and wide field imaging falloposcope for ovarian cancer detection. *Biomed Opt Express* 2017;**8**(1):124–36.

103. Flynn ER, Bryant HC. A biomagnetic system for in vivo cancer imaging. *Phys Med Biol* 2005;**50**(6):1273–93.

104. De Haro LP, Karaulanov T, Vreeland EC, *et al.* Magnetic relaxometry as applied to sensitive cancer detection and localization. *Biomed Tech* 2015;**60**(5):445–55.

105. Mathieu K, Lu Z, Yang H, et al. Feasibility of magnetic relaxometry for early ovarian cancer detection: preliminary evaluation ofsensitivity and specificity in cell culture and in mice [abstract]. In: *Proceedings of the 108th Annual Meeting of the American Association for Cancer Research 2017.* Philadelphia: AACR; 2017. Abstract nr 1864.

History of Cytoreductive Surgery in Ovarian Cancer Treatment

2

Alex A. Francoeur, Robert Bristow, and Jill Tseng

2.1 HISTORY OF PELVIC ADNEXAL SURGERY

To learn the history of anything, one must start at the beginning. The first operations on the ovaries were described by the Greek historian Athenaeus in ancient times where the ovaries of women were removed in parallel with the castration of men and to replace eunuchs (1). Ephraim McDowell is a more contemporary early account of a surgeon removing a large mass in the ovary. He encountered Jane Todd Crawford, a 46-year-old woman who was believed to be pregnant with twins but was found instead to have a large ovarian mass. Having never performed this surgery, he gave her a grim prognosis. In 1809,

DOI: 10.1201/9781003312475-2

on Christmas Day, without any modern anesthesia or antisepsis, he performed surgery on her in his kitchen. In his case report he describes his findings.

> The tumor appeared full in view but was so large we could not take it away entirely. We took out fifteen pounds of a dirty, gelatinous looking substance. After which we cut through the fallopian tube, and extracted the sac, which weighed seven pounds and one half (2).

He performed the surgery in an expeditious 25 minutes with no reported complications (3). The woman surprisingly lived to tell the tale, even outliving her surgeon, enjoying another 32 years of life.

2.2 THE BIRTH OF CYTOREDUCTION

The advent of a deeper understanding of cell and cancer biology as well as medical advancements in anesthesia and antisepsis ushered in a new frontier in knowledge and exploration of the management of ovarian tumors and cancer. Dr. Joe Meigs is long considered one of the fathers of gynecologic oncology. In 1934, he described a case series of 67 women with ovarian masses and cited the challenges in diagnosis and management due to lack of symptoms until advanced presentation (4). He reported a 5-year survival of 147 women following surgical management at a disappointing 16% (5). His insight for the time was quite accurate: "…treatment should consist of radical surgery…. If the omental cake can be removed successfully and easily, it too should be removed" (5). With the addition of x-ray therapy after surgery, Meigs reported an improvement in 5-year survival to 27%, the first description of adjuvant therapy after upfront primary surgery (6) (Figure 2.1).

Building off Dr. Meigs, a case series published in 1968 by Dr. Equinn William Munnell reported on 235 patients with ovarian cancer treated from 1952 to 1961 in New York. The surgeons performed exploratory laparotomies including total abdominal hysterectomy and bilateral salpingo-oophorectomy with attempts to remove all visible tumors including omentectomy, bowel surgery and upper abdominal surgery. They noted an improvement in 5-year survival to 27.5% with this more aggressive approach to surgical management (7).

A landmark trial in the history of primary debulking surgery was published in 1972 by Dr. C. Thomas Griffiths, a retrospective cohort of 60 cases of stage 2–3 ovarian cancer. This was the first study to demonstrate an inverse

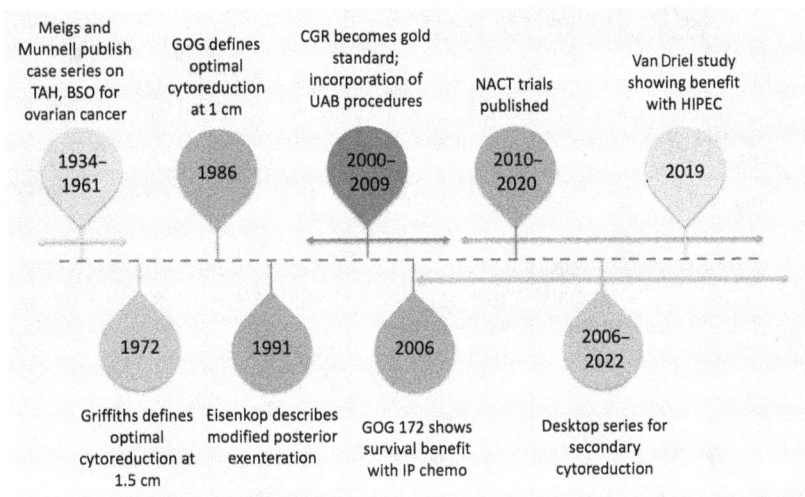

FIGURE 2.1   Timeline of the history of ovarian cancer. TAH, BSO = total abdominal hysterectomy, bilateral salpingo oophorectomy; GOG = Gynecologic Oncology Group; CGR = Complete gross residual; UAB = upper abdominal; IP = intraperitoneal; NACT = neoadjuvant chemotherapy; HIPEC = heated intraperitoneal chemotherapy.

correlation between residual tumor volume and overall patient survival (8). Additionally, he described the first case series of adjuvant chemotherapy, reporting that postoperative mustard therapy with radiation doubled survival time compared to radiation alone. He set the first cut off for residual disease after optimal cytoreduction at 1.5 cm, with a 5-year survival of 20% (9). Similar to Griffiths, Hacker et al. found an improvement in survival if residual disease was smaller than 1.5 cm. Hacker also reported a significant difference in survival with residual disease less than 0.5 cm compared to 0.5 to 1.5 cm (18 months vs. 40 months, respectively) (10). Griffith's study is the first time a disease volume was described, and it has further evolved over the years with the Gynecologic Oncology Group (GOG) defining optimal cytoreduction defined as no visible tumor greater than 1 cm left after surgery (11). Further studies examining the granularity of optimal cytoreduction found that the greatest survival benefit was seen in patients who were able to undergo surgery with resection to no gross residual disease (12–14).

A more recent meta-analysis by Bristow et al. in 2002 examined 81 studies and over 6,000 patients. The authors found that median overall survival with optimal cytoreduction was 36.8 months compared to 23.0 months in suboptimally debulked patients. They reported a rate of optimal cytoreduction of

75%. Additionally, they established the most important determinant of survival to be maximal cytoreduction. Their linear regression model demonstrated that each 10% increase in cytoreductive efforts led to a 5.5% increase in median survival time, thus setting forth a powerful argument for aiming towards no gross residual disease (Figure 2.2) (15). A study by du Bois et al. looking at pooled data from several randomized trials examined the impact of degree of cytoreduction in relation to patient outcome. They reported median survival in patients without any visible disease to be 99.1 months (95% CI, 83.5 — not reached), compared to 36.2 months (95% CI, 34.6–39.4) in patients with 1–10 mm of residual tumor, and 29.6 months (95% CI, 27.4–32.2) in patients with more than 10 mm residual disease (p < 0.0001). This held true when comparing stage at the time of surgery and histologic subtype (16).

Many surgical groups have reported improved survival outcomes with minimal additional morbidity in patients undergoing extensive cytoreductive surgery, strengthening the argument to push toward no gross residual disease (17–19). For example, Chi and colleagues from Memorial Sloan Kettering Cancer Center looked at a group of 465 women who underwent cytoreductive surgery for ovarian cancer. They found that median overall survival was 106 months with no visible disease, 66 months with 0.5 cm residual disease, 48 months with optimal cytoreduction (0.6–1 cm residual disease), 33 months with 1–2 cm residual disease and 34 months with greater than 2 cm residual disease, highlighting the absolute importance of optimal cytoreduction at the time of primary surgery (20).

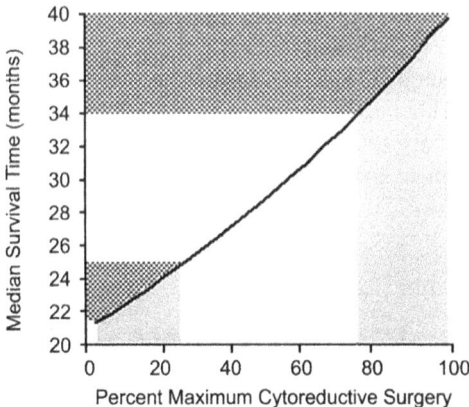

FIGURE 2.2 Simple linear regression analysis: de-logged median survival time plotted against percent maximal cytoreductive surgery. Gray area, maximal cytoreductive surgery 25% and > 75%; crosshatched area, corresponding range of median survival times. (from Ref. 15 with permission.)

Born out of the pursuit of complete cytoreductive efforts, many surgeons began pushing the boundaries in radical and upper abdominal surgery. Eisenkop described the modified posterior exenteration approach for a group of 47 patients in 1991, reporting a 38.3% complete cytoreduction rate, with morbidity and mortality rates of 19.1% and 2.1% respectively (21). Surgery to achieve no gross residual disease can require bowel resections in up to one third of patients, splenectomy in approximately 10% and urinary tract surgery in 3% (22). Harter et al. examined the role of lymphadenectomy in surgical cytoreduction in a randomized control trial. They found no difference in overall survival or progression-free survival with lymphadenectomy (overall survival: 69.2 months for no lymphadenectomy vs. 65.5 months with lymphadenectomy, HR 1.06, 95% CI 0.83–1.34, p = 0.65, progression-free survival: 25.5 months in both groups HR 1.11, 95% CI 0.92–1.34, p = 0.29). Complications, including repeat surgery and mortality within 60 days are higher in the lymphadenectomy group (23). Based on this, for normal lymph nodes, routine systematic lymphadenectomy in cytoreductive surgery is not recommended. If there is concern for lymphadenopathy on imaging or during intraoperative assessment, that node should be removed as part of the cytoreductive efforts.

Upper abdominal surgery can include surgery on the diaphragm, spleen, distal pancreas, gallbladder, liver and porta hepatis. Increasingly radical surgery in order to achieve no residual disease has been shown to improve patient overall survival (22). There comes a balance when considering these extensive surgeries to the patient population to which they are being offered; patients with ovarian cancer are in general older and may have multiple medical comorbidities. Performance status at the time of surgery is directly correlated with risk of morbidity (24). A systematic review reported 30-day mortality from primary debulking surgery to be 2.8% with 3-month all-cause mortality at 3.7 to 5.7% (25, 26). This rate has remained relatively constant over the last 30 years while complexity and extensiveness of surgery has increased. Furthermore, rates of complete gross resection, progression free and overall survival continued to improve (27).

2.3 MUSINGS IN ADJUVANT THERAPY

As mentioned in the previous section, the discovery of chemotherapy agents in the 1900s changed the way cancer could be targeted and treated. Dr. Griffiths first described adjuvant therapy in ovarian cancer, noting a survival benefit with the addition of mustard chemotherapy after surgery. Chemotherapy comes hand in hand with primary surgery for advanced ovarian cancer and a chapter on the history of cytoreductive surgery would be remiss not to go briefly into chemotherapy's history as well.

The rationale for chemotherapy after surgery is to induce cellular death in the remaining microscopic or macroscopic tumor cells to be able to obtain meaningful long-term survival or cure. In the late 1990s and early 2000s, GOG-111 and GOG-158 established adjuvant carboplatin and paclitaxel as standard of care for patients with advanced or aggressive epithelial ovarian cancer (28, 29). Different approaches to administration of adjuvant chemotherapy have been explored, most notably include studies examining intraperitoneal (IP) chemotherapy, the addition of bevacizumab to standard chemotherapy regimens and heated intraperitoneal chemotherapy (HIPEC).

IP chemotherapy is conceptually enticing as it provides a longer half-life of the chemotherapy agents and higher drug concentration in the peritoneal cavity where the majority of the tumor in ovarian cancer is located (30–34). In 1996, GOG-104 looked at adjuvant IV cyclophosphamide and cisplatin compared to IV cyclophosphamide and IP cisplatin, reporting an improvement in overall survival of 49 compared to 41 months with IP therapy (35). This was overshadowed by the results of GOG-111, moving the standard of care away from cyclophosphamide (28). In 2001, GOG-114 compared IV cisplatin and IV paclitaxel to IP cisplatin and IV paclitaxel and reported similar findings with improvement in progression-free survival from 22.2 months to 27.9 months, $p = 0.01$ (36). The findings of this trial were limited by toxicity events, preventing many patients in the IP group from receiving the allocated therapy. GOG-172, published in 2006 by Armstrong et al., compared IV and IP cisplatin in combination with IV paclitaxel as adjuvant therapy after optimal cytoreductive surgery. While the results in favor of IP chemotherapy were impressive with an increase in both progression free (median 23.8 vs. 18.3 months, $p = 0.027$) and overall survival (median 65.6 vs. 49.7 months, $p = 0.017$), the IP group was associated with significant toxicities. This included more myelosuppression, abdominal pain, IP catheter issues and bowel complications which led only 42% of patient's being able to complete all 6 cycles, limiting the ability to draw meaningful conclusions from this study (37). During the enrollment period of this study, GOG-158 was published and changed the standard of care chemotherapy from cisplatin and paclitaxel to carboplatin and paclitaxel, which also limits the generalizability of GOG-172 (29). It is clear that if toxicities of IP chemotherapy could be mitigated, IP chemotherapy would hold potential promise for benefit to patients.

Changes to the standard of care adjuvant therapy came in 2011 with the publication of GOG-218. This study was the first phase 3 randomized control trial adding bevacizumab, a vascular endothelial growth factor (VEGF) neutralizing monoclonal antibody, to standard of care chemotherapy. This study enrolled 1873 women worldwide with stage III (incompletely resected) or stage IV epithelial ovarian cancer. There were three groups: standard adjuvant chemotherapy using carboplatin and paclitaxel, carboplatin and paclitaxel plus bevacizumab starting in cycle 2 to 6, or carboplatin and paclitaxel with bevacizumab starting in cycle 2 for up to 22 cycles. The trial's primary endpoint, progression-free survival, was 4 months longer in the bevacizumab for up to 22 cycles cohort compared to the carboplatin- and paclitaxel-only group (14.1 vs. 10.3 months, HR 0.72; 95% CI, 0.63–0.82, p < 0.001). Higher rates of adverse effects were noted in the bevacizumab group, specifically rates of hypertension. There was no difference in overall survival in this study (38). A follow-up study of final survival data by Tewari et al. found no difference in overall survival in the prespecified study groups but a subgroup analysis demonstrated an overall survival benefit in patients with stage IV disease who received bevacizumab maintenance (42.9 vs. 32.6 months, HR 0.75; 95% CI, 0.59–0.95) (39).

Similar outcomes were reported in the European study ICON7. This study included patients with high-risk stage I and II disease in addition to stage III and IV disease. They found a 19% higher response rate in the bevacizumab group (67% vs. 48%) compared to standard chemotherapy. There was also a modest improvement in progression-free survival and overall survival, but in patients with high risk for progression (defined as FIGO stage IV disease or FIGO stage III disease with greater than 1 cm of residual disease after surgery), that effect was enhanced with PFS 14.5 months in the controls and 18.1 months with the addition of bevacizumab (p = 0.04) (HR for progression or death, 0.68; 95% CI, 0.55–0.85, p < 0.001). Overall survival was 28.8 and 36.6 months, respectively (40). This data indicates that bevacizumab has activity in high risk or distantly metastatic ovarian cancer and could be considered especially for stage IV patients or sub-optimally debulked patients as an adjunct to standard carboplatin and paclitaxel therapy.

GOG-252 attempted to further answer the question over the utility of IP chemotherapy in 2019, while building upon recent findings from GOG-218. The study had three arms: 1) IP carboplatin, IV paclitaxel and IV bevacizumab; 2) IP cisplatin, IV paclitaxel and IV bevacizumab; and 3) IV carboplatin, IV paclitaxel and IV bevacizumab. IP chemotherapy dosing was modified to try to improve patient compliance and toxicity that limited GOG-172. Patients all had stage II or higher ovarian cancer and were optimally resected. More patients were able to complete the IP regimen with reduced toxicity. Unfortunately, this was a negative study, with no difference in progression free or overall survival (41). For most gynecologic oncologists, this data signaled the end of IP chemotherapy although it is difficult to discern whether bevacizumab was a confounder or if this regimen is truly beneficial in an appropriately selected subset of patients. Currently, IP chemotherapy is uncommonly used in the United States.

Researchers then turned to HIPEC to see if outcomes could be improved with intraoperative hyperthermia to increase chemosensitivity and DNA damage (42–45). Van Driel et al. were the first to study this in a randomized phase 3 trial in 2018. Patients underwent 3 cycles of neoadjuvant chemotherapy (NACT) and were randomized to HIPEC with cisplatin ($100mg/m^2$) followed by adjuvant chemotherapy or standard adjuvant chemotherapy if cytoreduction was deemed to be optimal or without gross residual. In a cohort of 245 patients, median recurrence free survival was 14.2 months in the HIPEC group compared to 10.2 months in the standard of care group. They also found an increase in median overall survival with HIPEC (45.7 vs. 33.9 months, $p = 0.02$) (46). Since then, several smaller studies have found conflicting results and HIPEC remains hotly contested (47, 48). Critiques of the van Driel study include low patient numbers, as well as issues with accrual and imbalances in tumor histology in the treatment arms (49). There are no existing randomized trials looking at HIPEC during primary cytoreduction, however the international OVHIPEC-2 trial is currently accruing with data expected by 2026 (50). Other considerations include availability, cost and morbidity associated with HIPEC (51–53). Several other randomized trials are currently in process to help determine which patients, if any, would benefit most from this.

2.4 CHICKEN OR THE EGG: PRIMARY CYTOREDUCTION OR NEOADJUVANT CHEMOTHERAPY

One cannot discuss cytoreductive surgery for ovarian cancer without the elephant in the room—the debate over neoadjuvant chemotherapy or primary cytoreduction; which should come first? There are many physiologic advantages to cytoreductive surgery that could help improve the activity of adjuvant systemic chemotherapy. These include removal of resistant clones of tumor cells, creating a state of increased growth fraction as per the Gompertzian growth model, improved tumor perfusion, reduced drug resistance and increased immunogenicity response of the tumor (54–58). Secondary data analysis of GOG-52 and GOG-97 have shown no survival benefit in patients who undergo primary cytoreduction with greater than 2 cm residual tumor, highlighting the importance of residual tumor volume and ideally resection of all visible disease (59).

The goal then for NACT is to treat patients in whom optimal primary cytoreduction is deemed impossible with upfront chemotherapy followed by cytoreduction with the intent of achieving a more favorable surgical outcome. Vergote et al. published the first prospective, randomized, non-inferiority trial comparing NACT and primary debulking surgery followed by chemotherapy in 670 patients with stage IIIC or IV ovarian cancer. They found no difference in progression-free survival (29 months in primary surgery vs. 30 months in NACT) and found higher rates of optimal cytoreduction in the NACT arm. Patients had less mortality associated with NACT, with a reported postoperative death rate of 2.5% in the upfront surgery arm and 0.7% in the NACT arm. Rates of postoperative complications including hemorrhage, infection and venous complications were all lower in the NACT arm. Of note, the rate of optimal and complete cytoreduction were 41% and 20% in the upfront surgery arm, respectively. In a subgroup analysis comparing patients with no gross residual after upfront surgery compared to NACT, they found a lower overall survival in the NACT group (median OS 38 months in NACT vs. 45 months in primary surgery) (60). The CHORUS trial was another non-inferiority randomized control trial looking at the same question as Vergote et al. They noted similar findings with no difference in progression free or overall survival with a decrease in early mortality with NACT. They reported a higher rate of optimal debulking in the primary surgery arm, with a rate of 73% (61). Subsequently, a pooled analysis of results from Vergote et al. and the CHORUS trial was performed. In the combined population of 1200 patients, they found no difference in median progression-free survival when comparing primary surgery and NACT (27.6 months compared to 26.9 months, HR 0.97, 95% CI 0.86–1.09, p = 0.586). Additionally, they found that women with stage IV disease had improved outcomes with NACT instead of upfront surgery with a median progression-free survival 24.3 months compared to 21.2 months (HR 0.76, 95% CI 0.58–1.00, p = 0.048) (62). This highlights a potential group of patients that could most benefit from this approach to therapy in advanced ovarian cancer.

The Japan Clinical Oncology Group (JCOG0602) study was another randomized non-inferiority trial looking at NACT and upfront surgery. Optimal and complete cytoreduction rates were 37% and 12% respectively. They were unable to conclude that NACT was non-inferior to upfront surgery as there was no difference in progression-free survival in the groups and they did not meet their preset criteria for non-inferiority (15.1 months in upfront surgery and 16.4 months in NACT) (63). This was followed by the only inferiority designed randomized control trial. The SCORPION trial aimed to demonstrate that NACT was superior to upfront surgery. Patients all had a diagnostic laparoscopy to evaluate for high tumor burden and 171 total patients were randomized. This trial had a high rate of optimal cytoreduction at 92.8% and complete cytoreduction at 47.6%. Progression free and overall survival were not statistically different (14 and 43 months for NACT vs. 15 and 41 months for upfront surgery). There were much lower rates of major postoperative complications in the NACT group, 7.6% vs. 25.9%, and hospital stays were shorter in the NACT group (64).

There are extensively debated criticisms of the aforementioned trials and proponents for both approaches to management of primary ovarian cancer. The Vergote and JCOG trials were criticized for their low rate of optimal debulking compared to rates reported in the United States. Reported average time in the operating room was 180 minutes in Vergote et al. which is in contrast to other studies that quote average operating times over 300 minutes (27). There was no centralized method for defining complete resection; this was reported by the surgeon which allows for room for reporting bias. In general, their overall survival numbers were much lower than what had been routinely reported in prior trials, bringing the applicability of the results into question. The Vergote et al., CHORUS and JCOG trials were non-inferiority trials and as such do not indicate that NACT is superior to primary surgery. Additionally, the JCOG trial did not meet its non-inferiority endpoint either. SCORPION, the only designed superiority trial, failed to meet its preset criteria to make that judgment.

Based on the preceding data, it is important to be able to select the right patient for the right treatment. Those whose disease can be optimally resected should be considered for primary debulking surgery and those who cannot should be triaged to NACT. The challenge therein is in patient selection. Researchers have looked extensively at risk stratification with serum CA-125, imaging and diagnostic laparoscopy. While CA-125 levels and imaging can help the clinician predict burden of disease, they are poor at predicting the resectability of that disease. CA-125 levels greater than 500 U/ml generally predict higher burdens of disease but studies have found that it does not predict surgical outcomes, namely optimal cytoreduction rates. Chi et al. found that with CA-125 greater than 500 U/ml, upper abdominal procedures were required 50% of the time to reach optimal cytoreduction (65).

Imaging is a powerful modality to help identify ovarian tumors and the presence of metastatic disease. CT imaging is routinely obtained prior to treatment in ovarian cancer. CT can help identify metastasis that would not be amenable to primary resection such as central or multi-segmental parenchymal liver metastases, multiple parenchymal lung metastases, and brain metastases. Beyond that, studies report a low sensitivity in predicting which patients can be optimally cytoreduced, likely due to the fact that CT is not sensitive for detecting implants smaller than 5 mm (66, 67). Thus, imaging should always be used for preoperative planning but its use as the sole factor to determine the feasibility of an optimal cytoreductive surgical procedure should be limited.

Laparoscopy is another option that allows the surgeon to visually examine the abdomino-pelvic cavity to make a determination on resectability. Fagotti et al. created a scoring system assigning 0 or 2 points (present or absent) for the following categories: diaphragmatic disease, peritoneal carcinomatosis, mesenteric disease, omental disease, bowel infiltration, stomach infiltration and liver metastases. When the score was 8 or higher, there was zero probability of optimal cytoreduction (68). A Cochrane review looked at 18 studies and found a range of negative predictive values. They noted that only the study by Fagotti et al. avoided verification bias by performing laparotomy in all women. They reported a sensitivity of 0.95. The negative predictive value ranged from 0.69 to 1.00 for optimal debulking of less than 1 cm residual disease (69). This demonstrates that laparoscopy can be useful at identifying patients in whom cytoreduction is feasible but the adherence to preset criteria is important. Ultimately, even with defined criteria, the surgeon performing the procedure makes the final decision to proceed with or abort the procedure. Variations in training and surgical aggressiveness can change the way similar patients are managed.

The average age of diagnosis of ovarian cancer is 61, and with increasing age comes comorbidities and frailty. Patients with severe health conditions that compromise their performance status such as acute pulmonary embolism, decompensated heart failure or unstable angina should not undergo primary surgery. Nutritional status has been implicated as a factor portending a worse prognosis from surgery. One study found that patients with a prealbumin <10 mg/dl prior to surgery had a high rate of complications and mortality (61.5% and 23.1% respectively) (70). The same is true regarding albumin levels. Hypoalbuminemia predicts poor surgical outcomes as well as decreased survival (24 months vs. 83 months, p < 0.001) in one study after controlling for confounders (71). Increasing age can also be an independent factor for perioperative outcomes. Studies have shown that older women still have similar rates of optimal cytoreduction, but they are at higher risk of postoperative morbidity and mortality. One study of women 80 years and older reported an in-hospital mortality rate of 13% with limited ability to tolerate chemotherapy (72). The Mayo Clinic reported on outcomes of women older than 65 and found that the risk of complications increased with age but that if complete cytoreduction was achievable, patients saw similar survival benefits to younger patients. They identified preoperative albumin, ASA status and the presence of stage IV disease as the strongest risk factors for complications (73). Treatment planning in the elderly population must be carefully individualized as their performance status and comorbidities may vary widely, making management based oftentimes on best judgment. Care should be taken to fully assess patient comorbidities, nutritional status, social support and performance status prior to triaging them to primary surgery or NACT.

The debate between NACT and upfront surgery is nowhere near settled. There is also some concern that NACT may increase the rate of platinum resistance in the future in these patients, but this data is retrospective (74).

The decision for primary debulking or neoadjuvant chemotherapy rests on a high degree of judgment by the provider. The data is clear in terms of optimal cytoreduction and survival, but it is unclear regarding the route to achieve this. In general, if a patient can be optimally cytoreduced or debulked to no gross residual disease, and the patient has a good performance status, upfront surgery should be offered. The TRUST study, which is an international, prospective, inferiority design randomized control trial aimed at answering this question, finished recruitment in 2019 and data maturation should be available soon (75).

2.5 TO RE-DEBULK OR NOT? SECONDARY CYTOREDUCTION IN OVARIAN CANCER

In general, due to the advanced stage at diagnosis, patients undergoing cytoreductive surgery have a high rate of relapse, with up to 80% of patients having recurrent disease within two years, even with maximal surgical efforts (76). In the past, patients with recurrence were retreated with chemotherapy or offered palliative chemotherapy based on their platinum-sensitivity status. Since the early 2000s, smaller studies have reported survival benefit to secondary cytoreduction in recurrent platinum-sensitive ovarian cancer (77, 78). The DESKTOP series is the largest, most comprehensive set of studies to examine this question in depth.

The Eastern Cooperative Oncology Group (ECOG/AGO) published DESKTOP I in 2006. This was a retrospective cohort study of 256 patients who underwent cytoreductive surgery for recurrent ovarian cancer from 2000–2003. They found that only complete resection of all visible recurrent disease conferred a significant survival benefit. The median overall survival for complete gross resection was 45.2 months compared to 19.7 months with any residual disease (HR 3.71; 95% CI 2.27–6.05, p < 0.0001). Optimal cytoreduction with residual disease less than 1 cm was not associated with a survival benefit; only complete gross resection was oncologically advantageous. From this data, they were able to identify three factors highly associated with complete cytoreduction: early stage at initial diagnosis (FIGO I and II), no residual tumor after first cytoreductive surgery and ascites >500 ml. All of these factors combined were able to predict complete secondary cytoreduction in 79% of patients. From this, they created the Arbeitsgemeinschaft Gynäkologische Onkologie (AGO) score which is comprised of the presence of ascites, early stage of initial disease and an Eastern Cooperative Oncology Group (ECOG) performance status score of 0 (79).

The authors then set out to prospectively validate these findings. In the DESKTOP II study, patients with platinum-sensitive recurrence were scored per the AGO score and subsequent treatment with surgery versus chemotherapy was at the discretion of the oncologist. Of 516 patients with recurrence, 261 patients screened positive with the AGO score and were deemed likely to undergo complete surgical cytoreduction. 129 patients ultimately underwent secondary cytoreductive surgery and the rate of complete resection with no gross residual was 76%. These results were consistent with the findings in the DESKTOP I trial, validating the use of this score as a good predictor for resectability candidates (80).

This led to DESKTOP III, a multicenter randomized trial of patients with recurrent platinum-sensitive ovarian cancer undergoing secondary surgery followed by additional platinum chemotherapy versus standard chemotherapy alone. All patients were required to have a positive AGO score and the primary outcome was overall survival. They randomized 407 patients, of whom 75% in the surgery arm were able to be completely cytoreduced. Overall survival in the surgery group was 53.7 months compared to 46.0 months in the chemotherapy group (p = 0.02). Complete resection was associated with the greatest survival benefit; those patients had a median overall survival of 61.9 months. There was a 9% rate of surgical complications and no perioperative mortality reported (81).

Subsequently, two other randomized control trials have been published with data on secondary surgical cytoreduction. GOG-213, published in 2019, randomized patients with platinum-sensitive recurrence to secondary surgical cytoreduction followed by chemotherapy or upfront chemotherapy. The trial allowed providers to use bevacizumab at their discretion and unlike DESKTOP III, there were no preset criteria for determining resectability. They reported a complete surgical cytoreduction rate of 63%. There was no difference in progression free or overall survival between the groups (PFS 16.2 months in surgery group, 18.9 months in no surgery, HR 0.82 95% CI, 0.66 to 1.01, overall survival 50.6 months vs. 64.7 months, HR 1.29 95% CI 0.97 to 1.72) (82). The SOC-1 trial was a similarly designed trial in which 357 patients were randomized to surgery followed by chemotherapy or chemotherapy alone. Here, the authors used the iMODEL criteria and PET-CT imaging to select patients for surgery. The iMODEL score consists of initial FIGO stage, presence of residual disease from primary surgery, duration of platinum-free interval, ECOG status, CA-125 level at the time of recurrence and ascites present at the time of recurrence (83). They reported a complete resection rate of 77% and noted a significant difference in progression-free survival: with 17.4 months in the surgery group and 11.0 months in the no surgery group, p < 0.0001. Fully mature overall survival data is still pending (84).

The largest randomized control trials looking at secondary cytoreduction have yielded some incongruent results. DESKTOP III and SOC-1 were positive trials while GOG-213 was a negative trial. GOG-213 was the only trial to allow the use of bevacizumab which could have affected the results, similar to what was seen with IP chemotherapy in GOG-252. Additionally, DESKTOP and SOC-1 used validated selection models to determine which patients were highly likely to undergo complete cytoreduction of all visible disease, while GOG-213 did not use a pre-validated model and therefore possibly included patients who were unlikely to undergo complete cytoreduction. GOG-213 subsequently reported an approximately 10% lower rate of complete cytoreduction, which could have affected their findings. Overall, it appears that secondary cytoreduction for platinum-sensitive patients in whom complete gross resection of all disease is achievable can provide significant survival benefit. There are still unanswered questions regarding the addition of bevacizumab in this population. Additionally, these studies accrued prior to the publication of SOLO-1, and the widespread use of PARP–inhibitors may also affect patient outcomes, leaving more questions unanswered in regards to the management of patients with recurrence who are BRCA mutant or homologous recombination deficient (85). The SOC-3 trial (NCT03983226) aims to answer this question by administering niraparib maintenance in both surgery and no surgery groups (86).

2.6 A LITTLE LOOK OR WIDE OPEN? CHALLENGES TO SURGICAL APPROACH

Ovarian cancer cytoreductive surgery has classically been performed in an open approach. In order to completely explore the abdominopelvic cavity, one needs the tactile feedback and ability to move and retract organs that historically could only be achieved with an open incision. With the incorporation of NACT, more patients may have less disease burden at the time of interval cytoreductive surgery, thus potentially allowing for a minimally invasive approach. Several small studies have examined the utility of laparoscopic cytoreduction after NACT.

Brown and colleagues performed a retrospective study of patients who underwent traditional laparotomy compared to minimally invasive surgery after neoadjuvant chemotherapy. They reviewed 157 patients from 2006 to 2017, of which 53 underwent minimally invasive cytoreductive surgery and 104 underwent traditional laparotomy. They reported a conversion rate of 17%, with an additional 37% of patients who underwent a minimally invasive approach requiring a hand assist port or mini laparotomy. They reported a higher rate of R0 and optimal cytoreduction in the minimally invasive group (60.4% vs. 42.3% for R0 and 96.3% vs. 82.7% for optimal, p = 0.02). There was shorter hospital stay and less need for transfusion in the minimally invasive group, but they did have longer operating times. The median progression free (27 vs. 29 months, p = 0.45) and overall survival were not statistically different (37 vs. 35 months, p = 0.74) (87).

Another multicenter study looking at outcomes of minimally invasive surgery after NACT reported a case series of 127 patients. They reported 100% optimal cytoreduction with 96.1% to no gross residual tumor with the minimally invasive approach. Rate of conversion to laparotomy was reported as 3.9%. This group had a median progression-free survival of 23 months and a 5-year survival rate of 52% (88). While this is hypothesis generating data, the retrospective nature of both studies allows for a significant amount of selection bias. Additionally, with the previously discussed importance of reaching no gross residual for cytoreduction in ovarian cancer, it is concerning that the minimally invasive approach still had a fair number of patients that did not meet that benchmark. These patients may have benefited from an open surgical approach. A larger retrospective database study reported similar findings with no difference in 3-year overall survival between minimally invasive surgery and laparotomy (47.5% vs. 52.6%, p = 0.12) (89, 90).

There are some concerns with the minimally invasive approach. The aforementioned trials were not validation studies. To ensure complete cytoreduction, patients treated with a minimally invasive approach should then have undergone a laparotomy to confirm that the surgeons were successful but due to the retrospective nature of the studies, this was not possible. This brings into question whether the patient truly achieved a complete gross resection. There are regions in the abdomen that are challenging to access with the minimally invasive approach including Morrison's pouch, posterior diaphragm, posterior spleen, the lesser sac, porta hepatis and the caudate lobe of the liver. Future studies need to include documentation of these areas and should include confirmatory laparotomy.

The feasibility of minimally invasive cytoreductive surgery is being further investigated by the LANCE trial. They are accruing for a non-inferiority, prospective randomized trial for women who received NACT with complete or partial response with normalization of the CA-125. Their primary endpoint is progression-free survival and the study has been accruing since 2020 (91).

2.7 CONCLUSION

In conclusion, cytoreductive surgery for ovarian cancer has come a long way from its humble beginnings in Ephraim McDowell one Christmas morning. Surgeons are now performing more complex and extensive surgeries and extending patient life expectancy with advanced ovarian cancer with the help of improved adjuvant therapies. Medicine always has another frontier. There is much on the horizon in advanced ovarian cancer including the use of neoadjuvant chemotherapy, secondary cytoreduction and HIPEC. This review through history highlights the importance of well-designed, inclusive clinical trials to help provide the highest quality care for our patients.

REFERENCES

1. Clay C Observations on ovariotomy. *Boston Med Surg J* 1863; *69*:176–180.
2. McDowell E Three cases of extirpation of diseased ovaria. *Eclectic Repertory Anal Rev Med Philos.* 1817; *7*: 242–44.
3. Benigno BB, McDowell E, Todd Crawford J. The bicentennial of a surgical masterpiece. *Obstet Gynecol* 2009;*113*:1141–4.
4. Meigs JV, *Tumors of the Female Pelvic Organs*, MacMillan, New York, 1934.
5. Meigs JV, Cancer of the ovary, *N Engl J Med 220*(1939) 545–53.
6. Wheelock FC, Fennell Jr. RH, Meigs JV, Carcinoma of the ovary: Clinical and pathological evaluation, *N Engl J Med 245*(1951) 447–9.
7. Munnell EW. The changing prognosis and treatment in cancer of the ovary. A report of 235 patients with primary ovarian carcinoma 1952–1961. *Am J Obstet Gynecol* 1968;*100*(6):790–805.
8. Griffiths CT, Grogan RH, Hall TC, Advanced ovarian cancer: Primary treatment with surgery, radiotherapy, and chemotherapy, *Cancer 29*(1972):1–7.
9. Griffiths CT, Surgical resection of tumor bulk in the primary treatment of ovarian carcinoma, *Natl Cancer Inst Monogr 42*(1975) 101–4.
10. Whitney CW, Spirtos N, *Gynecologic Oncology Group Surgical Procedures Manual*, Gynecologic Oncology Group, Philadelphia, 2010.
11. Hacker NF, Berek JS, Lagasse LD, et al. Primary cytoreductive surgery for epithelial ovarian cancer. *Obstet Gynecol* 1983;*61*(4):413–20.
12. Winter III WE, Maxwell GL, Tian C, et al., Prognostic factors for stage III epithelial ovarian cancer: A Gynecologic Oncology Group Study, *J Clin Oncol 25*(2007):3621–27.
13. Chang SJ, Bristow RE, Evolution of surgical treatment paradigms for advanced stage ovarian cancer: Redefining 'optimal' residual disease, *Gynecol Oncol 125* (2012):(483–92.
14. Hamilton CA, Miller A, Casablanca T et al., Clinicopathologic characteristics associated with long-term survival in advanced epithelial ovarian cancer: An NRG Oncology/Gynecologic Oncology Group ancillary data study, *Gynecol Oncol* (2018);*148*(2):275–80.
15. Bristow RE, Tomacruz RS, Armstrong DK et al. Survival effect of maximal cytoreductive surgery for advanced ovarian carcinoma during the platinum era: A meta-analysis. *J Clin Oncol.* 2002;*20*(5):1248–59. Corrected and republished in: J Clin Oncol. 2023;*41*(25):4065–4076.

16. du Bois A, Reuss A, Pujade-Lauraine E, et al. Role of surgical outcome as prognostic factor in advanced epithelial ovarian cancer: A combined exploratory analysis of 3 prospectively randomized phase 3 multicenter trials: By the Arbeitsgemeinschaft Gynaekologische Onkologie Studiengruppe Ovarialkarzinom (AGO-OVAR) and the Groupe d'Investigateurs Nationaux Pour les Etudes des Cancers de l'Ovaire (GINECO). *Cancer* 2009;*115*(6):1234–44.

17. Aletti GD, Dowdy SC, Gostout BS et al., Quality improvement in the surgical approach to advanced ovarian cancer: The Mayo Clinic experience, *J Am Coll Surg 208*(2009):614–20.

18. Chi DS, Eisenhauer EL, Zivanovic O et al., Improved progression-free and overall survival in advanced ovarian cancer as a result of a change in surgical paradigm, *Gynecol Oncol 114*(2009):26–31.

19. Harter P, Muallem ZM, Buhrmann C et al., Impact of a structured quality management program on surgical outcome in primary advanced ovarian cancer, *Gynecol Oncol 121*(2011):615–9.

20. Chi DS, Eisenhauer EL, Lang J, et al. What is the optimal goal of primary cytoreductive surgery for bulky stage IIIC epithelial ovarian carcinoma (EOC)? *Gynecol Oncol* 2006;*103*(2):559–64.

21. Eisenkop SM, Nalick RH, Teng NN. Modified posterior exenteration for ovarian cancer. *Obstet Gynecol* 1991;*78*(5 Pt 1):879–85.

22. Eisenhauer EL, Abu-Rustum NR, Sonoda Y, et al. The addition of extensive upper abdominal surgery to achieve optimal cytoreduction improves survival in patients with stages IIIC-IV epithelial ovarian cancer. *Gynecol Oncol* 2006; *103*(3):1083–90.

23. Harter P, Sehouli J, Lorusso D, et al. A Randomized Trial of Lymphadenectomy in Patients with Advanced Ovarian Neoplasms. *N Engl J Med* 2019;*380*(9):822–32.

24. Gerestein CG, Nieuwenhuyzen-de Boer GM, Eijkemans MJ, et al. Prediction of 30-day morbidity after primary cytoreductive surgery for advanced stage ovarian cancer. *Eur J Cancer* 2010;*46*(1):102–9.

25. Aletti GD, Santillan A, Eisenhauer EL, et al. A new frontier for quality of care in gynecologic oncology surgery: Multi-institutional assessment of short-term outcomes for ovarian cancer using a risk-adjusted model. *Gynecol Oncol* 2007;*107*(1):99–106.

26. Gerestein CG, Damhuis RA, Burger CW, et al. Postoperative mortality after primary cytoreductive surgery for advanced stage epithelial ovarian cancer: A systematic review. *Gynecol Oncol* 2009;*114*(3):523–7.

27. Tseng JH, Cowan RA, Zhou Q, et al. Continuous improvement in primary Debulking surgery for advanced ovarian cancer: Do increased complete gross resection rates independently lead to increased progression-free and overall survival? *Gynecol Oncol* 2018;*151*(1):24–31.

28. McGuire WP, Hoskins WJ, Brady MF, et al. Cyclophosphamide and cisplatin compared with paclitaxel and cisplatin in patients with stage III and stage IV ovarian cancer. *N Engl J Med* 1996;334:1–6.

29. Ozols RF, Bundy BN, Fowler J, et al. Randomized phase III study of cisplatin (CIS)/paclitaxel (PAC) versus carboplatin (CARBO)/PAC in optinal stage III epithelial ovarian cancer (OC): A Gynecologic Oncology Group trial (GOG-158). *Proc Am Soc Clin Oncol* 1999; *18*:356a (abstract 1373).

30. Dedrick RL, Myers CE, Bungay PM et al. Pharmacokinetic rationale for peritoneal drug administration in the treatment of ovarian cancer. *Cancer Treat Rep* 1978;*62*:111.
31. Cannistra SA. Cancer of the ovary. *N Engl J Med* 2004:*351*:2519–29.
32. Thigpen T. The if and when of surgical debulking for ovarian carcinoma. *N Engl J Med* 2004;*351*:2544–6.
33. Markman M. Intraperitoneal antineoplastic agents for tumors principally confined to the peritoneal cavity. *Cancer Treat Rev* 1986;*13*:219–42.
34. Markman F, Francis P, Rowinsky E et al. Intraperitoneal paclitaxel: A possible role in the management of ovarian cancer? *Semin Oncol* 1995;*22*:84–7
35. Alberts DS, Liu PY, Hannigan EV et al. Intraperitoneal cisplatin plus intravenous cyclophosphamide versus intravenous cisplatin plus intravenous cyclophosphamide for stage III ovarian cancer. *N Engl J Med* 1996;*335*:1950–5.
36. Markman M, Bundy BN, Alberts DS, et al. Phase III trial of standard-dose intravenous cisplatin plus paclitaxel versus moderately high-dose carboplatin followed by intravenous paclitaxel and intraperitoneal cisplatin in small-volume stage III ovarian carcinoma: An intergroup study of the Gynecologic Oncology Group, Southwestern Oncology Group, and Eastern Cooperative Oncology Group. *J Clin Oncol* 2001;*19*(4):1001–7.
37. Armstrong DK, Bundy B, Wenzel L, et al; Gynecologic Oncology Group. Intraperitoneal cisplatin and paclitaxel in ovarian cancer. *N Engl J Med* 2006;*354*(1):34–43.
38. Burger RA, Brady MF, Bookman MA, et al; Gynecologic Oncology Group. Incorporation of bevacizumab in the primary treatment of ovarian cancer. *N Engl J Med* 2011;*365*(26):2473–83.
39. Tewari KS, Burger RA, Enserro D, et al. Final overall survival of a randomized trial of bevacizumab for primary treatment of ovarian cancer. *J Clin Oncol* 2019;*37*(26):2317–28.
40. Perren TJ, Swart AM, Pfisterer J, et al; ICON7 Investigators. A phase 3 trial of bevacizumab in ovarian cancer. *N Engl J Med.* 2011;*365*(26):2484–96.
41. Walker JL, Brady MF, Wenzel L, et al. Randomized trial of intravenous versus intraperitoneal chemotherapy plus bevacizumab in advanced ovarian carcinoma: An NRG oncology/gynecologic oncology group study. *J Clin Oncol.* 2019;*37*(16):1380–90.
42. Zivanovic O, Abramian A, Kullmann M, et al. s. *Int J Cancer* 2015;*136*(3): 699–708.
43. Los G, van Vugt MJ, den Engelse L, et al. Effects of temperature on the interaction of cisplatin and carboplatin with cellular DNA *Biochem Pharmacol* 1993;*46*(7):1229–37.
44. Los G, van Vugt MJ, Pinedo HM. Response of peritoneal solid tumours after intraperitoneal chemohyperthermia treatment with cisplatin or carboplatin, *Br J Cancer* 1994;*69*(2):235–41.
45. Los G, Verdegaal E, Noteborn H.P.J.M., et al. Cellular pharmacokinetics of carboplatin and cisplatin in relation to their cytotoxic action, *Biochem Pharmacol* 1991;*42*(2):357–63.
46. van Driel WJ, Koole SN, Sikorska K et al. Hyperthermic intraperitoneal chemotherapy in ovarian cancer. *N Engl J Med* 2018;*378*(3):230–40.

47. Antonio CCP, Alida GG, Elena GG, et al. Cytoreductive surgery with or without HIPEC after neoadjuvant chemotherapy in ovarian cancer: A phase 3 clinical trial. *Ann Surg Oncol* 2022;*29*(4):2617–25.
48. Lim MC, Chang SJ, Park B, et al; HIPEC for ovarian cancer collaborators. Survival after hyperthermic intraperitoneal chemotherapy and primary or interval cytoreductive surgery in ovarian cancer: A randomized clinical trial. *JAMA Surg* 2022;*157*(5):374–83.
49. Vergote I, Harter P, Chiva L. Hyperthermic intraperitoneal chemotherapy does not improve survival in advanced ovarian cancer. *Cancer* 2019;*125* Suppl 24:4594–7.
50. Koole S, van Stein R, Sikorska K et al., Primary cytoreductive surgery with or without hyperthermic intraperitoneal chemotherapy (HIPEC) for FIGO stage III epithelial ovarian cancer: OVHIPEC-2, a phase III randomized clinical trial. *Int J Gynecol Cancer 30*(2020):888–92.
51. Koole SN, Kieffer JM, Sikorska K et al., Health-related quality of life after interval cytoreductive surgery with or without hyperthermic intraperitoneal chemotherapy (HIPEC) in patients with stage III ovarian cancer. *Eur J Surg Oncol* (2019);*47*(1):101–7.
52. Behbakht K, Cohn DE, Straughn JM, Hyperthermic intraperitoneal chemotherapy (HIPEC) is cost-effective in the management of primary ovarian cancer. *Gynecol Oncol 151*(2018):4–5.
53. Lim SL, Havrilesky LJ, Habib AS et al. Cost-effectiveness of hyperthermic intraperitoneal chemotherapy (HIPEC) at interval debulking of epithelial ovarian cancer following neoadjuvant chemotherapy. *Gynecol Oncol 153*(2019):376–80.
54. Goldie JH, Coldman AJ. A mathematic model for relating the drug sensitivity of tumors to their spontaneous mutation rate. *Cancer Treat Rep* 1979;*63*(11–12):1727–33.
55. Gunduz N, Fisher B, Saffer EA. Effect of surgical removal on the growth and kinetics of residual tumor. *Cancer Re* 1979;*39*:3861–3865.
56. DeVita VT. The relationship between tumor mass and resistance to chemotherapy. Implications for surgical adjuvant treatment of cancer. *Cancer* 1983;*51*:1209–20
57. Skipper HE. Adjuvant chemotherapy. *Cancer* 1978;*41*:936–40.
58. Bookman MA, Berek JS. Biologic and immunologic therapy of ovarian cancer. *Hematol Oncol Clin North Am* 1992;*6*:941–65.
59. Hoskins WJ, McGuire WP, Brady MF, et al. The effect of diameter of largest residual disease on survival after primary cytoreductive surgery in patients with suboptimal residual epithelial ovarian carcinoma. *Am J Obstet Gynecol* 1994;*170*(4):974–9; discussion 979–80.
60. Vergote I, Tropé CG, Amant F, et al; European organization for research and treatment of cancer-gynaecological cancer group; NCIC clinical trials group. Neoadjuvant chemotherapy or primary surgery in stage IIIC or IV ovarian cancer. *N Engl J Med* 2010;*363*(10):943–53.
61. Kehoe S, Hook J, Nankivell M, et al. Primary chemotherapy versus primary surgery for newly diagnosed advanced ovarian cancer (CHORUS): An open-label, randomised, controlled, non-inferiority trial. *Lancet* 2015;*386*(9990):249–57.
62. Vergote I, Coens C, Nankivell M, et al; EORTC; MRC CHORUS study investigators. Neoadjuvant chemotherapy versus debulking surgery in advanced tubo-ovarian cancers: Pooled analysis of individual patient data from the EORTC 55971 and CHORUS trials. *Lancet Oncol.* 2018;*19*(12):1680–87.

63. Onda T, Satoh T, Saito T, et al; Japan Clinical Oncology Group. Comparison of treatment invasiveness between upfront debulking surgery versus interval debulking surgery following neoadjuvant chemotherapy for stage III/IV ovarian, tubal, and peritoneal cancers in a phase III randomized trial: Japan Clinical Oncology Group Study JCOG0602. *Eur J Cancer* 2016;*64*:22–31.

64. Fagotti A, Ferrandina MG, Vizzielli G, et al. Randomized trial of primary debulking surgery versus neoadjuvant chemotherapy for advanced epithelial ovarian cancer (SCORPION-NCT01461850). *Int J Gynecol Cancer* 2020;*30*(11): 1657–64.

65. Chi DS, Zivanovic O, Palayekar MJ, et al. A contemporary analysis of the ability of preoperative serum CA–125 to predict primary cytoreductive outcome in patients with advanced ovarian, tubal and peritoneal carcinoma. *Gynecol Oncol* 2009;*112*(1):6–10.

66. Nasser S, Lazaridis A, Evangelou M, et al. Correlation of pre-operative CT findings with surgical & histological tumor dissemination patterns at cytoreduction for primary advanced and relapsed epithelial ovarian cancer: A retrospective evaluation. *Gynecol Oncol* 2016;*143*(2):264–9.

67. Koh JL, Yan TD, Glenn D, et al. Evaluation of preoperative computed tomography in estimating peritoneal cancer index in colorectal peritoneal carcinomatosis. *Ann Surg Oncol* 2009;*16*(2):327–33.

68. Fagotti A, Ferrandina G, Fanfani F, et al. Prospective validation of a laparoscopic predictive model for optimal cytoreduction in advanced ovarian carcinoma. *Am J Obstet Gynecol* 2008;*199*(6):642.e1–6.

69. van de Vrie R, Rutten MJ, Asseler JD, et al. Laparoscopy for diagnosing resectability of disease in women with advanced ovarian cancer. *Cochrane Database Syst Rev* 2019, 3. *CD009786*.

70. Geisler JP, Linnemeier GC, Thomas AJ, et al. Nutritional assessment using prealbumin as an objective criterion to determine whom should not undergo primary radical cytoreductive surgery for ovarian cancer. *Gynecol Oncol* 2007;*106*(1):128–31.

71. Ataseven B, du Bois A, Reinthaller A, et al. Pre-operative serum albumin is associated with post-operative complication rate and overall survival in patients with epithelial ovarian cancer undergoing cytoreductive surgery. *Gynecol Oncol* 2015;*138*(3):560–5.

72. Moore KN, Reid MS, Fong DN, et al. Ovarian cancer in the octogenarian: Does the paradigm of aggressive cytoreductive surgery and chemotherapy still apply? *Gynecol Oncol* 2008;*110*(2):133–9.

73. Langstraat C, Aletti GD, Cliby WA. Morbidity, mortality and overall survival in elderly women undergoing primary surgical debulking for ovarian cancer: A delicate balance requiring individualization. *Gynecol Oncol* 2011;*123*: 187–91.

74. Rauh-Hain JA, Nitschmann CC, Worley MJ Jr, et al. Platinum resistance after neoadjuvant chemotherapy compared to primary surgery in patients with advanced epithelial ovarian carcinoma. *Gynecol Oncol* 2013;*129*(1):63–8.

75. Reuss A, du Bois A, Harter P, et al. TRUST: Trial of Radical Upfront Surgical Therapy in advanced ovarian cancer (ENGOT ov33/AGO-OVAR OP7). *Int J Gynecol Cancer* 2019;*29*(8):1327–31.

76. Agarwal R, Kaye SB. Ovarian cancer: Strategies for overcoming resistance to chemotherapy. *Nat Rev Cancer* 2003;*3*(7):502–16.

77. Munkarah A, Levenback C, Wolf JK, et al. Secondary cytoreductive surgery for localized intra-abdominal recurrences in epithelial ovarian cancer. *Gynecol Oncol* 2001;*81*(2):237–41.

78. Bristow RE, Puri I, Chi DS. Cytoreductive surgery for recurrent ovarian cancer: A meta-analysis. *Gynecol Oncol* 2009;*112*(1):265–74.

79. Harter P, du Bois A, Hahmann M, et al; Arbeitsgemeinschaft Gynaekologische Onkologie Ovarian Committee; AGO Ovarian Cancer Study Group. Surgery in recurrent ovarian cancer: The Arbeitsgemeinschaft Gynaekologische Onkologie (AGO) DESKTOP OVAR trial. *Ann Surg Oncol* 2006;*13*(12):1702–10.

80. Harter P, Sehouli J, Reuss A, et al. Prospective validation study of a predictive score for operability of recurrent ovarian cancer: The Multicenter Intergroup Study DESKTOP II. A project of the AGO Kommission OVAR, AGO Study Group, NOGGO, AGO-Austria, and MITO. *Int J Gynecol Cancer* 2011;*21*(2): 289–95.

81. Harter P, Sehouli J, Vergote I, et al; DESKTOP III investigators. Randomized trial of cytoreductive surgery for relapsed ovarian cancer. *N Engl J Med* 2021;*385*(23):2123–31. Erratum in: *N Engl J Med.* 2022;386(7):704.

82. Coleman RL, Spirtos NM, Enserro D, et al. Secondary surgical cytoreduction for recurrent ovarian cancer. *N Engl J Med* 2019 Nov 14;*381*(20):1929–39.

83. Tian WJ, Chi DS, Sehouli J, et al. A risk model for secondary cytoreductive surgery in recurrent ovarian cancer: An evidence-based proposal for patient selection. *Ann Surg Oncol* 2012 Feb;*19*(2):597–604.

84. Shi T, Zhu J, Feng Y, et al. Secondary cytoreduction followed by chemotherapy versus chemotherapy alone in platinum-sensitive relapsed ovarian cancer (SOC–1): A multicentre, open-label, randomised, phase 3 trial. *Lancet Oncol* 2021 Apr;*22*(4):439–49.

85. Moore K, Colombo N, Scambia G, et al. Maintenance olaparib in patients with newly diagnosed advanced ovarian cancer. *N Engl J Med* 2018 Dec 27;*379*(26):2495–505.

86. Shi T, Yin S, Zhu J, et al. A phase II trial of cytoreductive surgery combined with niraparib maintenance in platinum-sensitive, secondary recurrent ovarian cancer: SGOG SOC–3 study. *J Gynecol Oncol* 2020;*31*(3):e61. Erratum in: *J Gynecol Oncol.* 2022 Jul;33(4):e63.

87. Brown J, Drury L, Crane EK, et al. When less is more: Minimally invasive surgery compared with laparotomy for interval debulking after neoadjuvant chemotherapy in women with advanced ovarian cancer. *J Minim Invasive Gynecol* 2019;*26*(5):902–9.

88. Fagotti A, Gueli Alletti S, Corrado G, et al. The International Mission study: Minimally invasive surgery in ovarian neoplasms after neoadjuvant chemotherapy. *Int J Gynecol Cancer* 2019;*29*(1):5–9.

89. Melamed A, Nitecki R, Boruta DM, et al. Laparoscopy compared with laparotomy for debulking ovarian cancer after neoadjuvant chemotherapy. *Obstet Gynecol* 2017;*129*(5):861–9

90. Jorgensen K, Melamed A, Wu CF, et al. Minimally invasive interval debulking surgery for advanced ovarian cancer after neoadjuvant chemotherapy. *Gynecol Oncol* 2023;*172*:130–137.

91. Nitecki R, Rauh-Hain JA, Melamed A, et al. Laparoscopic cytoreduction After Neoadjuvant ChEmotherapy (LANCE). *Int J Gynecol Cancer* 2020;*30*(9): 1450–4.

Hereditary Breast and Ovarian Cancer

3

A Historical Perspective

Payal D. Shah and Susan M. Domchek

3.1 ORIGINS OF THE CONCEPT OF GENETIC CANCER SUSCEPTIBILITY

For hundreds of years, it has been observed that certain families have a preponderance of cancer, while cancer remains a rare event in others. In many families with a high prevalence of cancer, members are diagnosed with one of a few, characteristic cancer types, often at younger ages than would be expected, and often with evidence of vertical transmission of cancer risk. In the 1600s, after observing breast cancer in members of the same household, Holland physicians Zacutus Lusitani[1] and Nicholas Tulp[2] independently concluded that cancers were contagious; their monographs[3] were published in 1649 (Lusitani) and 1652 (Tulp) and the physicians recommended isolation of cancer patients as a mode of cancer prevention. Some throughout the 17th and 18th centuries continued to hold this belief.

DOI: 10.1201/9781003312475-3

The fundamental laws of the science of modern genetics were published in 1866 by Gregor Mendel.[4] He discussed segregation of "unit-characters," one character dominant and the other recessive, and published his well-known garden pea plant (*Pisum sativum*) hybridization experiments that gave rise to a greater understanding of heredity and of a biological basis for the transmission of traits from parents to offspring.

In 1866, the French physician Pierre Paul Broca published a two-volume treatise entitled Traite des Tumeurs;[5-7] this work represented a departure from the theory that cancer was contagious and instead supported the concept of cancer inheritance. Inspired by his wife who, like many of her family members was afflicted by breast cancer at an early age, Dr. Broca created a four-generation pedigree of the family of "Mrs. Z." He noted that a daughter may be born long before her mother and maternal grandmother developed breast cancer, and that the daughter may still, herself, develop it many years later. Broca wrote

> a person in whom are assembled unknown conditions, which expose him to later become cancerous, can transmit to his posterity this group of conditions before they have even manifested themselves in him. Also, having received the diathesis from one of his forebears, he may escape, during a long and healthy life, the consequences of that hereditary state, and may pass on to his children the disease from which he was spared.

In what is essentially an early description of genetic predisposition with incomplete penetrance and variable expressivity, Broca shifted the focus toward an unidentified causative agent passed down from generation to generation. He noted, "a remarkable fact about the inheritance of cancer is the perfect health which is enjoyed for many years by persons who carry the 'germ' of this illness." He postulated that the cause of disease lay dormant in a given individual, inactive in the body for an indefinite period of time, and then became active and caused the disease.

William Bateson was an English biologist and early proponent of Mendel's ideas. In 1905, Bateson wrote a letter to a colleague[8] proposing that the term "genetics" be used to designate "the study of heredity." The term "gene" was coined in 1909 by Danish botanist Wilhelm Johannsen to describe the Mendelian units of heredity,[9] who also distinguished genotype, genetic traits, from phenotype, the outward manifestation of those traits. These terms are felt to have etymological origins from the Greek word γένος (genos), meaning "kin, birth," or γενεά (genea) meaning "generation, race."

In 1912, Isaac Levin at Columbia University College of Physicians and Surgeons published "The influence of heredity on cancer" and noted: "The question presents itself as to whether it is feasible to suppose a priori that the occurrence of cancer may also be influenced by heredity." He describes a combination of three factors that cause cancer:

> a direct cause – the nature of which is as yet unknown, and which may be a group of cells changed biologically so that it has become capable of unlimited proliferation -, plus a mediate cause, which may be an injury or a changed mode of living or any other environmental condition, - and plus an intrinsic constitutional susceptibility.

Importantly, Levin also noted organ specificity in terms of localization of the cancers occurring within a family.[10]

The following year, Aldred Scott Warthin reported on the "cancer family syndrome" and updated this report throughout the twentieth century.[11,12] He reported on Family G, a family with multiple cases of uterine cancer, stomach cancer, intestinal cancer and "cancer of the abdomen." Foretelling modern-day cancer genetics principles, he discussed the importance of relying on pathology or "morbidity" reports rather than on less-precise mortality reports when conducting epidemiological studies to understand familial cancer risk, and he discussed the inadequacy of obtaining an incomplete family history from a patient.

In parallel to this increased recognition of the heritability of cancer, a better understanding of the structure and composition of genes was occurring. American geneticist and 1933 Nobel Prize winner Thomas Hunt Morgan described the linear arrangement of genes on chromosomes, a theory he expanded upon in his book, *Mechanism of Mendelian Heredity* published in 1915.[13] The structure of DNA was elucidated later, by James Watson, Francis Crick and Rosalind Franklin in 1953.[14] These discoveries enabled scientists to look deeply at affected families in an effort to identify causative genes.

In this context, Henry T. Lynch noted familial cancer prevalence in multiple reports including that of Family N.[15] In 1974, noting "cancer-prone lines" of the family, Lynch reported that

> pedigree analyses repeatedly showed that individuals from particular lineages tend to develop cancers of specific anatomic sites. It is suggested that gene-transmitted constitutional differences may interact with nongenetic factors, possibly oncogenic viruses, to produce cancer in such family members who are at relatively high risk.

Like Levin, Lynch noted the presence of a causative factor that was intrinsic and inherited, as well as the impact of the external environment. He furthermore had the foresight to advocate for "cancer control programs… for better management of these familial cancer problems." Lynch later published family histories of cancer from an oncology clinic and noted the incomplete inclusion of family history in medical charts, advocating for more thorough inquiries and reporting of family history to improve care.[16,17]

Later in the 20th century, there were at least two notable factors propelling forward the modern field of cancer genetics. First, the potential for a distinct alteration in a gene to directly cause disease became clear. Huntington's disease is a rare, adult-onset, autosomal dominant neurodegenerative disease that had been known for over a hundred years to have familial transmission. In 1983, the Huntington (*HTT*) gene was molecularly mapped to chromosome 4p16.3,[18] followed by the DNA sequencing of this gene in 1993[19] allowing the precise nature of the mutation to be elucidated: in patients with Huntington's disease, the *HTT* gene contains an abnormal number of CAG nucleotide repeats. Second, multiple observational and epidemiological studies continued to repeatedly demonstrate that the risk of certain cancers was increased in individuals with family histories of these cancers.[15,17,20–22] These seminal studies contributed to an early understanding of Li-Fraumeni syndrome[23,24] and Lynch syndrome[17] in the late 1980s and 1990s. A preponderance of breast and other cancers including ovarian cancer was noted and was actively being investigated. A hereditary basis for ovarian cancer specifically was, at this time, relatively underrepresented in the literature.

3.2 RACE TO FIND THE "BREAST CANCER GENE"

In January 1974, Dr. Mary-Claire King was hired by Dr. Nicholas Petrakis as a researcher at the University of California, San Francisco to study the genetics of breast cancer.[25–27] Dr. King and colleagues conducted complex segregation analyses to evaluate patterns of breast cancer occurrence in 1579 families from the National Cancer Institute's Surveillance, Epidemiology and End Results (SEER) program. This seminal work published in 1988 concluded that an autosomal dominant, highly penetrant susceptibility gene explained observed disease clustering.[27] Researchers next focused on finding the gene, i.e., mapping the gene to a physical location on a chromosome. This step required worldwide collaboration to develop a genetic map, the first iteration of which was conceived of in 1987.[28,29] Mapping the breast cancer gene involved an approach termed linkage analysis, in which many markers were genotyped in individuals considered informative, in this case, individuals with personal and/or family histories of breast cancer. The 173rd marker tested in Dr. King's laboratory, D17S74, was a variable number of tandem repeat (VNTR) marker on position

21 of the long arm of chromosome 17 (17q21).[30] Using predefined model-based linkage parameters, this marker was felt to be linked with 10^6:1 odds to 7 families with an average age of breast cancer onset ≤ 45 years, and demonstrated no linkage with families demonstrating late-onset disease. These landmark data were published in *Science* in 1990; the location of a highly penetrant breast cancer gene had been mapped. In this same year, the Human Genome Project launched in the United States. One year later, Myriad Genetics was founded.

Determining the chromosomal locale of the breast cancer gene was a critical step to more precisely determine the physical location of the gene because it allowed the region of interest to be reduced to a manageable size – 17q21, identified as the chromosomal locale of interest in 1990, was 22Mb. The focus thus shifted to positional cloning and study of potential mutations disabling the gene. Multiple research teams at universities, in government and in industry attempted to narrow down the location of the breast cancer gene,[31–35] named *"BRCA1"* by Dr. King in 1991. The media nicknamed this competition "The Race." Dr. King and colleagues at Berkeley partnered with Francis Collins first at the University of Michigan and then at the NIH, Anne Bowcock and colleagues at the University of Texas Southwestern Medical Center, and Jeffrey Boyd at the National Institute of Environmental Health Sciences. Dr. King notes, "we were four groups in five towns in three time zones, keeping in contact without Internet or cell phones. It seemed normal at the time."[26] Dr. Mark Skolnick and colleagues at Myriad Genetics were among those in "The Race." At the same time that positional cloning attempts were ongoing, data emerged demonstrating that the breast cancer susceptibility gene on chromosome 17q was also associated with a predisposition to hereditary ovarian cancer.[36] Ultimately, in 1994, Dr. Skolnick and colleagues were the first to complete and publish positional cloning data identifying *BRCA1*, understood by that time to be a breast and ovarian cancer susceptibility gene.[37] By this time, competition was so strong that the article submitted to *Science* intentionally omitted the DNA sequence, added only at the time of publication.[25] On September 15, 1994, the news of the cloning of *BRCA1* was featured on the front page of the *New York Times* described as "capturing a genetic trophy so ferociously coveted and loudly heralded that it had taken on a near-mythic aura."[38]

Following the discovery of *BRCA1*, numerous questions remained including but not limited to the biological function of the encoded protein; why a gene with ubiquitous expression has organ site-specific variability in cancer risks; and what additional factors may explain hereditary cancer risk in the absence of *BRCA1*. The Breast Cancer Linkage Consortium (BCLC) was founded in 1989 as a worldwide data-sharing platform aimed at addressing many of these questions and published early studies quantifying breast and ovarian cancer risk[39].

3.3 FINDING BRCA2

In April 1995, a group of British researchers gathered in a London restaurant.[40] Among them was Dr. Alan Ashworth, then at the Chester Beatty Laboratory, who proclaimed, on a paper napkin smudged with chocolate ice-cream, that the *BRCA2* gene would be cloned, likely by him, within the next 12 months and that the successful researcher would be responsible for buying all others dinner. The paper napkin was initialed by half-a-dozen "witnesses", i.e., colleagues around the table.

Dr. Ashworth's prediction was accurate. In September 1994, concurrent with the announcement of the *BRCA1* gene sequence, the chromosomal mapping of *BRCA2* to chromosome 13q12-13 was published.[41] Co-authors included Mark Skolnick, David Goldgar and researchers from the University of Utah, as well as a number of other academic researchers from Europe and the United States. Amidst *BRCA1* gene patent disputes discussed later, this group that had collaboratively published the location of the *BRCA2* gene divided into competing groups working to sequence the gene. The sequence was first published in December 1995 by British researchers, including Dr. Ashworth.[42] However, in the same month shortly before the article was published, Myriad announced that it had also sequenced the gene, entered this data into GenBank and had filed for a patent. Myriad authors published their report on the *BRCA2* gene sequence in March 1996.[43]

3.4 BRCA1 AND BRCA2 PATENTS

Shortly after the biotechnology firm Myriad Genetics cloned *BRCA1* in 1994, the company developed medical tests to detect mutations in *BRCA1* and *BRCA2*. Such testing involved separating segments of DNA containing the nucleotide sequences of interest and creating a complementary DNA (cDNA) strand which contains only exons. Based on Myriad's assertion that it was the first company to discover the precise location and sequence of *BRCA1* and *BRCA2*, Myriad successfully obtained patents on the acts of isolating the genes and synthesizing cDNA. At the time, the University of Pennsylvania was partial owner of some *BRCA2* patents licensed by Myriad. A separate company, OncorMed, had also been issued patents for a full-length coding sequence of the *BRCA1* gene and also received a worldwide, exclusive license to the *BRCA2* gene.[44] After mutual lawsuits for patent infringement, Myriad ultimately acquired OncorMed's *BRCA1/2* testing business and patent rights in 1998. Thus, by the end of the 1990s, Myriad had consolidated control over substantially all U.S. patent rights for *BRCA1* and *BRCA2*.

The result of these patents was that Myriad held sole power to conduct medical *BRCA1* and *BRCA2* testing for which it charged as much as $4040 per test.[45] From 1996 through 2013, Myriad performed over one million tests for *BRCA1* and *BRCA2* and generated over $2.8 billion in revenues;[46] the ability of other groups to carry out genetic testing of patients was substantially limited. The patents were a subject of dispute almost immediately. One point of contention related to two NIH researchers who co-authored the article cloning *BRCA1* but were not listed as coinventors on the patents;[47] the NIH was thus denied a share of royalties from testing. Peter Meldrum, president of Myriad at the time, justified this, stating that the NIH researchers had made no unique contribution to the discovery. Many in the research community and women's health groups were similarly concerned about Myriad's patents. Fran Visco, president of the advocacy organization National Breast Cancer Coalition, noted "Women gave their blood for this research. I know many of these women, and they didn't give blood so some company could make millions of dollars."

In 2013, the Supreme Court unanimously overturned Myriad's patents relating to *BRCA1* and *BRCA2*, noting in their ruling of *Association for Molecular Pathology et al. v. Myriad Genetics, Inc. et al.*, that while cDNA is subject to patent, human genes are products of nature and therefore "are not patent eligible subject matter.[48]" The nullification of this patent occurred alongside key technological advances in genetic testing. Early germline testing entailed the time-intensive process of gene-by-gene Sanger sequencing; massively parallel sequencing[49] replaced Sanger sequencing around the time of the Myriad patent loss. Massively parallel sequencing enabled high-throughput testing of multiple genes in less time and at a lower cost than Sanger sequencing; furthermore, it allowed for greater identification of large genomic rearrangements including clinically relevant rearrangements in *BRCA1* and *BRCA2* that were not easily detected by Sanger sequencing methods. The overall result was a competitive market with multiple companies offering multigene panel testing. The cost of clinical genetic testing dropped dramatically, leading to its broader accessibility.

3.5 EVOLUTION OF GENETIC TESTING

The first commercial test for mutations in the *BRCA1* and *BRCA2* genes was brought to market in 1996.[50] Conversations about identification of appropriate candidates for testing, clinical validity, clinical utility, regulation of testing, cost of testing, clinical implications, the potential for discrimination on the basis of test results, invasion of privacy and social and psychological issues began immediately.[51-59] One author noted, "the ground is shifting almost from week to week." The American Society of Clinical Oncology (ASCO) put forth a statement on genetic testing for cancer susceptibility in May 1996[60] advocating for clinical family history assessment, participation in prospective studies or registries, education for health professionals, consent for germline testing, pre- and post-test counselling and testing only in high-risk individuals in whom the tests can be interpreted and acted upon. ASCO also endorsed regulatory requirements for laboratories, legislation prohibiting discrimination, programs to enhance access to care and patient-oriented research to evaluate psychological consequences of genetic testing. In response to these guidelines, an ad hoc task force created a resource document for cancer genetics education curriculum development.[61] The National Institutes of Health (NIH) and the Department of Energy Working Group on Ethical, Legal, and Social Implications of Human Genome Research, or ELSI, established a Task Force on Genetic Testing to help put forth guidelines for genetic testing implementation which were published in 1997.[62] In sum, guidelines and literature at the time highlighted the limitations in knowledge and the need for further research. Despite extensive discussions, optimal implementation of testing programs in the context of complex medical, ethical and legal questions remained murky.

In the earliest years of germline testing, candidates for such testing were identified on the basis of a personal and/or family history suggestive of an inherited cancer syndrome. Testing involved Sanger sequencing, often restricted to *BRCA1* and *BRCA2*, followed by additional phenotype-directed testing of a limited number of high penetrance genes associated with specific syndromes, such as *TP53* (Li Fraumeni Syndrome) and *PTEN* (Cowden syndrome) if initial testing was negative. If a patient reported Ashkenazi Jewish ancestry, initial testing of *BRCA1* and *BRCA2* often included only the three founder mutations[63] *BRCA1* 185delAG (c.68_69delAG [p.Glu23Valfs]); *BRCA1* 5382insC (c.5266dupC [p.Gln1756Profs]) and *BRCA2*6174delT (c.5946delT [p.Ser-1982Argfs]), rather than sequencing of the full genes. Myriad, still the only company performing clinical testing at this time due to patents, initially offered *BRCA1* and *BRCA2* full gene sequencing through comprehensive BRACAnalysis; however it was widely known that up to 10% of mutations in *BRCA1* and *BRCA2* were missed by this type of testing including large genomic rearrangements.[64] In 2002, Myriad began to offer testing for the five most common large genomic rearrangements and on July 31, 2006, Myriad began offering a separate test called the BRACAnalysis large rearrangement test (BART) to detect some of these missed mutations. BART was a separate test with a separate cost of up to $700 with variable insurance coverage.[65] Many appropriate candidates for large rearrangement evaluation were therefore not having such testing done. The 2013 National Comprehensive Cancer Network updated guidelines supporting large rearrangement testing for all patients undergoing testing, and insurance approval of such testing broadened as well.[66] Myriad Genetics began incorporating large rearrangement testing into routine *BRCA1* and *BRCA2* testing through integrated BRACAnalysis.[67]

Myriad lost its patent on the *BRCA1* and *BRCA2* genes on June 13, 2013; on the day of this ruling, Ambry Genetics and Gene by Gene both announced that they were offering *BRCA1* and *BRCA2* testing. Multiple other genetic testing companies including GeneDX, Ambry Genetics, Invitae, Color Genomics, Labcorp and others followed suit shortly thereafter. These initial years after patent loss were highly competitive.

There were multiple consequences of the shift from a monopoly to a competitive market for hereditary breast and ovarian cancer testing. There was clear economic impact: the cost of testing decreased. Access to testing accordingly improved. Access to genetic data and data sharing was also transformed; many testing companies contributed data to the publicly available NIH database, ClinVar.[68] Scientists and physicians also launched the BRCA Exchange,[69] an online database of BRCA variants from multiple sources, which had representatives from many of the large genetic testing companies. During these same years, the technologies for DNA sequencing as well as for accumulating, digitizing, storing and analyzing genetic data evolved tremendously. The marked technological advances alongside greater access to genetic testing (generating larger datasets) and improved data sharing efforts propelled forward tremendous advances in patient care.

3.6 GENETIC INFORMATION NONDISCRIMINATION ACT OF 2008

In the 1990s, as genetic testing for inherited cancer susceptibility became a reality, concerns grew about discrimination on the basis of test results.[70-72] Fear of such discrimination could and undoubtedly did prevent individuals from undergoing genetic testing, even in cases in which the results of such testing could substantially impact the care of individuals and their family members. Furthermore, fear of discrimination deterred individuals from participating in genetic research.[70] Bills aiming to prevent such discrimination were introduced into the legislature as early as 1995. At the time, sequencing of the human genome was just beginning and a limited number of genetic tests were available; many believed legislation addressing genetic discrimination was premature.[73] Ultimately, on May 21, 2008, President George W. Bush signed the Genetic Information Nondiscrimination Act of 2008 (GINA) to provide protection to American citizens from discrimination based on their genetic information in both health insurance (Title I) and employment (Title II).

Title I specifically prevents health insurance companies from using genetic information to determine insurance eligibility or to make decisions regarding insurance coverage, underwriting or premium-setting. Health insurance companies may not request or require individuals to undergo genetic testing or to provide genetic information including family medical history, family members' diagnoses and family members' genetic test results. These protections extend to private health insurers, Medicare, Medicaid, Federal Employees Health Benefits and the Veterans Health Administration.

Title II of GINA prevents employers from using genetic information to inform decisions such as hiring, firing, promotions, pay and job assignments. Employers and certain employment-related entities such as employment agencies, labor organizations and others cannot require or request genetic information and/or testing as a condition of employment.

There are important nuances and exceptions to GINA protections. The Title I health insurance protections do not cover long-term care insurance, life insurance or disability insurance, although some state laws have additional protections that address these gaps. They do not extend to the U.S. military; although the U.S. military's TRICARE insurance program does prevent the use of genetic information for coverage, underwriting and premium-setting, TRICARE is available only to those employed by the U.S. military and the U.S. military *is* permitted to use genetic and medical information to make employment decisions. Notably, GINA also does not apply to employers with fewer than 15 employees. Furthermore, under GINA, employers are permitted to request employees' genetic information for the purposes of voluntary wellness programs, but they are not permitted to reward employees for doing so nor can they penalize employees for withholding genetic information.

GINA is enforced by the Department of Health and Human Services, the Department of Labor, the Department of Treasury and the Equal Opportunity Employment Commission. GINA is felt to have favorably impacted genetic research by alleviating participants' concerns about discrimination due to results. Compliance with GINA requires that informed consent forms for clinical research involving genetics include information on risks and a description of the measures being taken to ensure confidentiality of records.

3.7 THE GENETIC LANDSCAPE OF OVARIAN CANCER RISK AND MITIGATION STRATEGIES

It was and remains widely known that *BRCA1* and *BRCA2* genes are associated with hereditary breast and ovarian cancers. Precise estimates vary and may be quite dependent on family history and other modifiers,[74–76] but *BRCA1* is associated with a markedly elevated (50–80%) lifetime risk of breast cancer; 20–45% lifetime risk of ovarian cancer, as well as elevated risks of pancreas and prostate cancer. *BRCA2* is also associated with elevated lifetime risks of breast (40–60%) and ovarian (10–20%) cancers, as well as elevated risks of prostate cancer, pancreas cancer and male breast cancer. As multigene panel testing became more widespread, additional genes emerged as being associated with ovarian cancer. These included genes involved in Lynch Syndrome, specifically *MSH2*, *EPCAM*, *MLH1* and to a lesser degree, *MSH6*; *RAD51C*; *RAD51D*; *BRIP1*; *PALB2* and *ATM*. The lifetime risk of ovarian cancer with a pathogenic variant in a Lynch Syndrome gene varies substantially based on gene and population ascertained in the literature, but is approximately 4–20% for *MLH1*, 8–38% for *MSH2* and *EPCAM*, and slightly elevated above population risk for *MSH6*.[77] Other genes with elevated lifetime risks of high-grade serous ovarian cancer are: *RAD51C*[78] and *RAD51D*[79,80] (10–15%); *BRIP1*[81–84] (5–15%); *ATM* [85,86] (3–5%) and *PALB2*[87–89] (3–5%).

The most effective and well-studied ovarian cancer risk reduction strategy available is the use of oral contraceptive pills (OCP).[90–92] Oral contraceptive use is associated with a duration-dependent reduction in the risk of ovarian cancer. The risk reduction is quantified at approximately 5% per year of use, and about 50% for ≥ 10 years of use. The favorable effect of OCP against ovarian cancer risk persists for more than 30 years after the completion of use. This risk is weighed against a potential increase in breast cancer risk. Counselling *BRCA1/2* carriers considering OCP use warrants a balanced discussion of risks and benefits as well as individualized consideration of prior risk-reducing surgeries, prior breast cancer, age and patient preferences.[93] In 2017, it became clear that high-grade serous ovarian carcinoma often originates in the fallopian tubes;[94] tubal ligation was studied and was found to also reduce ovarian cancer risk.[93] Ongoing studies are investigating whether salpingectomy with delayed oophorectomy (in order to minimize the impact of early menopause) is safe and effective.[95] Effective ovarian cancer screening for early detection of disease has been elusive and the use of CA-125 blood testing with transvaginal ultrasound is therefore not universally recommended for women at high risk.

Because of the mortality associated with high-grade serous ovarian cancer and lack of early detection strategies, individuals with *BRCA1* and *BRCA2* pathogenic variants are advised to undergo risk reducing salpingo-oophorectomy at approximately age 35–40 (*BRCA1*) or 40–45 (*BRCA2*), after the completion of childbearing goals. Data suggest that risk-reducing salpingo-oophorectomy in *BRCA1* and *BRCA2* carriers may not only reduce risk of ovarian cancer but may also reduce ovarian cancer-specific, breast cancer-specific and all-cause mortality.[96–98] Based on these data, risk-reducing salpingo-oophorectomy is recommended for those with pathogenic variants in other moderate- or high-risk ovarian cancer susceptibility genes including *BRIP1*, *RAD51C*, *RAD51D* and others. Given that ovarian cancer precursor lesions develop in the fallopian tubes and that oophorectomy has undesired consequences, ongoing research is evaluating salpingectomy as a prevention strategy. The aforementioned risk mitigation and prevention strategies represent important examples of learning from those at highest risk and extrapolating findings to others with elevated ovarian cancer risk, with risk determined largely on the basis of germline alterations.

3.8 THE DEVELOPMENT OF GENETICALLY TARGETED OVARIAN CANCER THERAPEUTICS

An understanding of the biology of *BRCA1*- and *BRCA2*-associated ovarian cancers led to the development of targeted inhibitors of poly-ADP-ribose polymerase (PARPi). The development of PARPi was not only transformative for patients with *BRCA1/2*-associated ovarian cancer, but it was groundbreaking for non-*BRCA1/2*-associated ovarian cancer as well as *BRCA1*- and *BRCA2*-associated cancers more broadly. The original scientific premise for PARPi activity in tumors associated with *BRCA1* or *BRCA2* was the concept of synthetic lethality: a highly specific PARP inhibitor induces a DNA lesion and a tumor-restricted genetic loss of function for homologous recombination, the DNA repair pathway required to repair the original lesion. Since that time, the understanding of the biological basis for response and resistance to PARPi has markedly evolved. Early clinical trials of the PARP inhibitor olaparib[99–101] demonstrated tolerability and efficacy that correlated with platinum sensitivity. In 2014, on the basis of promising phase II data,[102] olaparib obtained accelerated FDA approval for the treatment of women with *BRCA1*- or

BRCA2-associated advanced ovarian cancer following treatment with three or more prior lines of chemotherapy.[103] As discussed in more depth in the essay dedicated to PARPi, subsequent studies led to the full FDA approval of olaparib for patients with ovarian cancer as well as FDA approvals of niraparib and rucaparib for patients with advanced ovarian cancer in multiple contexts,[104] including within and outside of a germline *BRCA1* or *BRCA2* mutation: treatment of recurrent disease, maintenance therapy in platinum-sensitive recurrent disease and maintenance therapy in platinum-sensitive primary disease.[105] Early successes seen with treating ovarian cancer patients with PARPi provided impetus for study of PARPi in ovarian cancer more broadly and for patients with other *BRCA1/2*- associated or homologous recombination deficiency-associated cancers.

3.9 CONCLUSION

The current understanding of hereditary breast and ovarian cancer pathology and management is a product of hundreds of years of scientific inquiry including clinical and laboratory research. It is now known that the *BRCA1* and *BRCA2* genes are drivers of hereditary breast and ovarian cancer syndrome, but alterations in additional genes can also increase the risk of breast and/or ovarian cancers, with Lynch Syndrome genes, *RAD51C*, *RAD51D*, *BRIP1*, *PALB2* and *ATM* being among those that carry elevated risks of ovarian cancer. The journey to reach this current understanding was fraught with industry collaborations that were both strained and productive. Psychosocial, ethical and legal issues compelled deep consideration of the optimal approach to implementation and care delivery. However, this journey ultimately paved the way for the development of risk mitigation and therapeutic strategies that have had a transformative impact on patients and families, indeed improving survival of patients with ovarian cancer. Many of the lessons learned from the study of *BRCA1* and *BRCA2* have informed prevention and treatment strategies more broadly, including in patients with sporadic or other inherited forms of ovarian cancer as well as breast, prostate and pancreas cancers. Perhaps most important to keep in mind as the field moves forward is that none of the preceding advancements would have been possible to achieve without patient participation in research. Further developments and innovations in the field of hereditary breast and ovarian cancer syndrome will only occur with patients as key partners in this work. See further Figure 3.1.

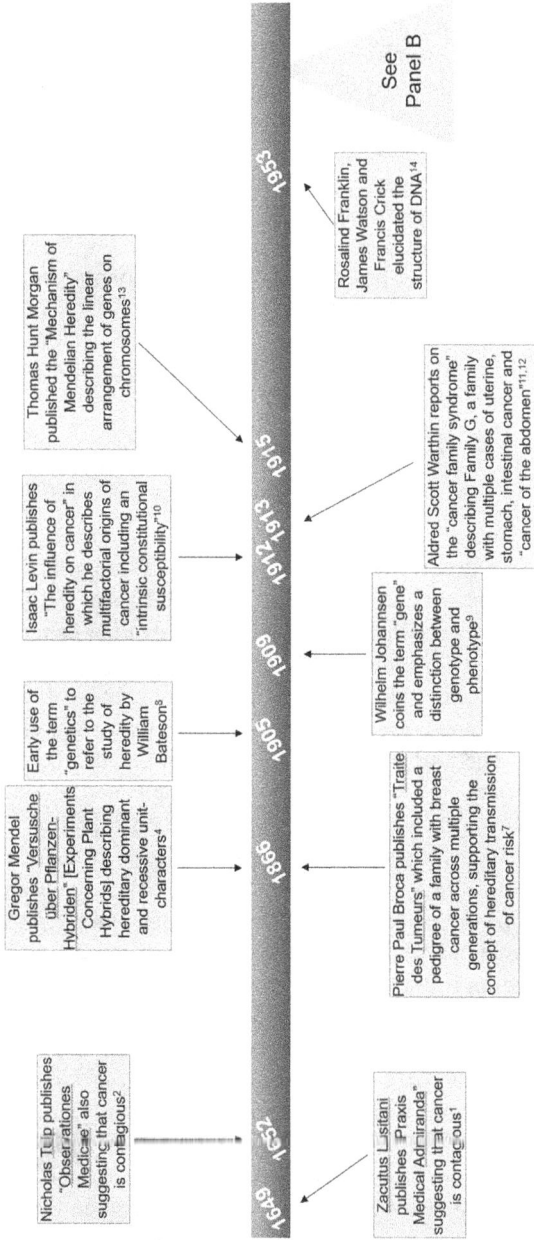

Nicholas Tulp publishes "Observationes Medicae" also suggesting that cancer is contagious[2]

Zacutus Lusitani publishes "Praxis Medical Admiranda" suggesting that cancer is contagious[1]

Gregor Mendel publishes "Versusche über Pflanzen-Hybriden" [Experiments Concerning Plant Hybrids] describing hereditary dominant and recessive unit-characters[4]

Early use of the term "genetics" to refer to the study of heredity by William Bateson[8]

Isaac Levin publishes "The influence of heredity on cancer" in which he describes multifactorial origins of cancer including an "intrinsic constitutional susceptibility"[10]

Thomas Hunt Morgan published the "Mechanism of Mendelian Heredity" describing the linear arrangement of genes on chromosomes[13]

Pierre Paul Broca publishes "Traite des Tumeurs" which included a pedigree of a family with breast cancer across multiple generations, supporting the concept of hereditary transmission of cancer risk[7]

Wilhelm Johannsen coins the term "gene" and emphasizes a distinction between genotype and phenotype[9]

Aldred Scott Warthin reports on the "cancer family syndrome" describing Family G, a family with multiple cases of uterine, stomach, intestinal cancer and "cancer of the abdomen"[11,12]

Rosalind Franklin, James Watson and Francis Crick elucidated the structure of DNA[14]

See Panel B

1649 1652 1866 1905 1909 1912 1913 1915 1953

(a)

FIGURE 3.1   Major historical events in hereditary breast and ovarian cancer, from the 1600s through the elucidation of DNA structure (a) and from the mapping of BRCA1 through 2020

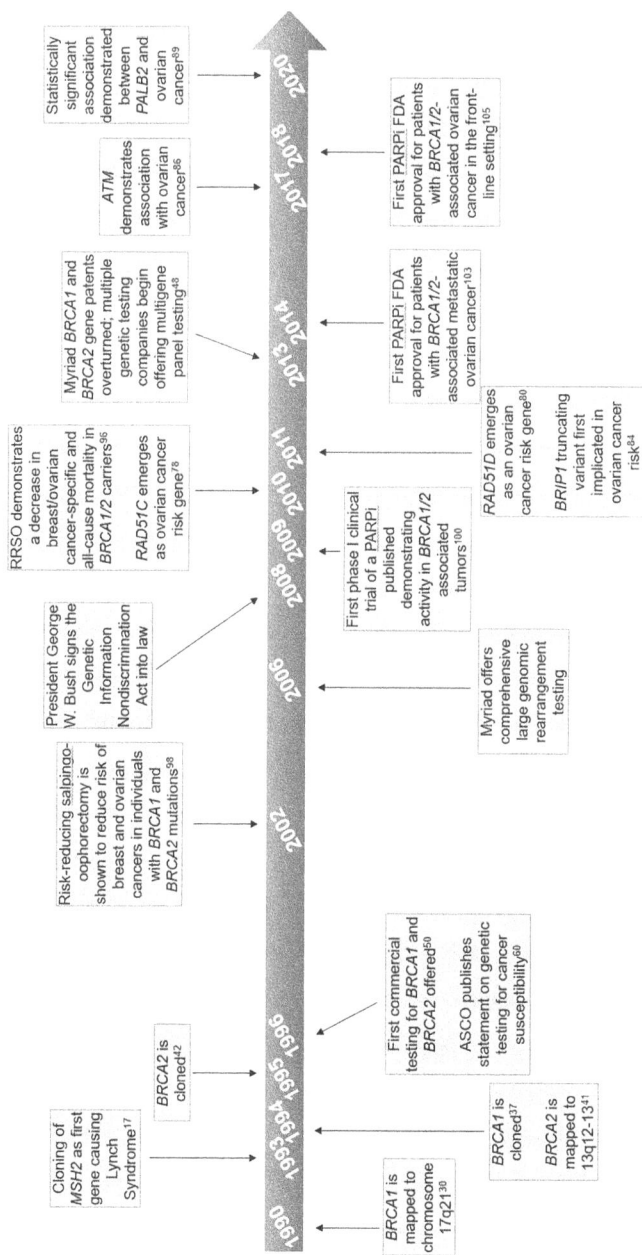

FIGURE 3.1   (Continued) (b). This timeline includes key events in hereditary breast and ovarian cancer from the discovery of major causative genes to landmark advances in risk mitigation and therapeutics. Of note, only the first PARPi approvals in the recurrent and frontline settings are included.

REFERENCES

1. Lusitani Z: *Praxis Medical Admiranda.* Lugduni: J. Hugvetan, 1649.
2. Tulp N: *Observationes Medicae.* Amstelredami: Elzevirium, 1652.
3. Hajdu SI: A note from history: landmarks in history of cancer, part 2. *Cancer 117*:2811–20, 2011.
4. Zhang H, Chen W, Sun K: Mendelism: New insights from Gregor Mendel's Lectures in Brno. *Genetics 207*:1–8, 2017.
5. Krush AJ: Contributions of Pierre Paul Broca to Cancer Genetics. Transactions of the Nebraska Academy of Sciences VII, 1979.
6. van der Groep P, van der Wall E, van Diest PJ: Pathology of hereditary breast cancer. *Cell Oncol (Dordr) 34*:71–88, 2011.
7. Broca PP: *Traite des Tumeurs.* 1866.
8. Szabo AT, Poczai P: The emergence of genetics from Festetics' sheep through Mendel's peas to Bateson's chickens. *J Genet 98*, 2019.
9. Johannsen W: *Elemente der exakten Erblichkeitslehre.* Jena: Gustav Fischer, 1909.
10. Levin I: The influence of heredity on cancer. *Zeitschrift für Krebsforschung 11*:547–58, 1912.
11. Warthin AS: Heredity with reference to carcinoma. *Archives of Internal Medicine 12*:546–55, 1913.
12. Douglas JA, Gruber SB, Meister KA, et al: History and molecular genetics of Lynch syndrome in family G: a century later. *JAMA 294*:2195–202, 2005.
13. Morgan TH: *The mechanism of Mendelian heredity.* New York: Henry Holt and Company, 1915.
14. Watson JD, Crick FH: Molecular structure of nucleic acids: a structure for deoxyribose nucleic acid. *Nature, 4356* April 25, 1953. Nature *248*:765, 1974.
15. Lynch HT: Familial cancer prevalence spanning eight years. *Family N. Archives of Internal Medicine 134* 5:931–8, 1974.
16. Lynch HT, Follett KL, Lynch PM, et al: Family history in an oncology clinic. Implications for cancer genetics. *JAMA 242*:1268–72, 1979.
17. Lynch HT, Snyder CL, Shaw TG, et al: Milestones of Lynch syndrome: 1895–2015. *Nat Rev Cancer 15*:181–94, 2015.
18. Gusella JF, Wexler NS, Conneally PM, et al: A polymorphic DNA marker genetically linked to Huntington's disease. *Nature 306*:234–8, 1983.
19. MacDonald M.E.A.C., Duyao MP, Myers RH, et al: A novel gene containing a trinucleotide repeat that is expanded and unstable on Huntington's disease chromosomes. The Huntington's Disease Collaborative Research Group. *Cell 72*:971–83, 1993.
20. Haagensen CD: Family history of breast carcinoma in women predisposed to develop breast carcinoma. *J Natl Cancer Inst 48*:1025–7, 1972.
21. Huis J, Dausset J: Letter: Identical malignant diseases in members of the same family. *Nouv Presse Med 3*:1237, 1974.
22. Morgan RW, Vakil DV, Chipman ML: Breast feeding, family history, and breast disease. *Am J Epidemiol 99*:117–22, 1974.
23. Li FP, Fraumeni JF, Jr., Mulvihill JJ, et al: A cancer family syndrome in twenty-four kindreds. *Cancer Res 48*:5358–62, 1988.

24. Blattner WA, McGuire DB, Mulvihill JJ, et al: Genealogy of cancer in a family. *JAMA 241*:259–61, 1979.

25. Dalpe R, Bouchard L, Houle AJ, et al: Watching the race to find the breast cancer genes. *Sci Technol Human Values 28*:187–216, 2003.

26. King MC: "The race" to clone BRCA1. *Science 343*:1462–5, 2014.

27. Newman B, Austin MA, Lee M, et al: Inheritance of human breast cancer: evidence for autosomal dominant transmission in high-risk families. *Proc Natl Acad Sci U S A 85*:3044–8, 1988.

28. Smith L, Hood L: Mapping and sequencing the human genome: How to proceed. *Bio/Technology 5*:933–9, 1987.

29. *Mapping and Sequencing the Human Genome.* Washington (DC), 1988.

30. Hall JM, Lee MK, Newman B, et al: Linkage of early-onset familial breast cancer to chromosome 17q21. *Science 250*:1684–9, 1990.

31. Chamberlain JS, Boehnke M, Frank TS, et al: BRCA1 maps proximal to D17S579 on chromosome 17q21 by genetic analysis. *Am J Hum Genet 52*:792–8, 1993.

32. Feunteun J, Narod SA, Lynch HT, et al: A breast-ovarian cancer susceptibility gene maps to chromosome 17q21. *Am J Hum Genet 52*:736–42, 1993.

33. Tonin P, Serova O, Simard J, et al: The gene for hereditary breast-ovarian cancer, BRCA1, maps distal to EDH17B2 in chromosome region 17q12-q21. *Hum Mol Genet 3*:1679–82, 1994.

34. Bowcock AM, Anderson LA, Friedman LS, et al: THRA1 and D17S183 flank an interval of < 4 cM for the breast-ovarian cancer gene (BRCA1) on chromosome 17q21. *Am J Hum Genet 52*:718–22, 1993.

35. Hall JM, Friedman L, Guenther C, et al: Closing in on a breast cancer gene on chromosome 17q. *Am J Hum Genet 50*:1235–42, 1992.

36. Narod SA, Feunteun J, Lynch HT, et al: Familial breast-ovarian cancer locus on chromosome 17q12-q23. *Lancet 338*:82–3, 1991.

37. Miki Y, Swensen J, Shattuck-Eidens D, et al: A strong candidate for the breast and ovarian cancer susceptibility gene BRCA1. *Science 266*:66–71, 1994.

38. Angier N: Scientists identify a mutant gene tied to hereditary breast cancer, *The New York Times*, 1994, pp 1.

39. Easton DF, Bishop DT, Ford D, et al: Genetic linkage analysis in familial breast and ovarian cancer: results from 214 families. The breast cancer linkage consortium. *Am J Hum Genet 52*:678–701, 1993.

40. Touching base: April fool. *Nature Genetics 12*:354, 1996.

41. Wooster R, Neuhausen SL, Mangion J, et al: Localization of a breast cancer susceptibility gene, BRCA2, to chromosome 13q12–13. *Science 265*:2088–90, 1994.

42. Wooster R, Bignell G, Lancaster J, et al: Identification of the breast cancer susceptibility gene BRCA2. *Nature 378*:789–92, 1995.

43. Tavtigian SV, Simard J, Rommens J, et al: The complete BRCA2 gene and mutations in chromosome 13q-linked kindreds. *Nat Genet 12*:333–7, 1996.

44. *Writers BHEM: Oncormed Issued Patent for BRCA1 Gene.* Bloomberg, 1997.

45. Cartwright-Smith L: Patenting genes: what does Association for Molecular Pathology v. Myriad Genetics mean for genetic testing and research? *Public Health Rep 129*:289–92, 2014.

46. Cook-Deegan R, Niehaus A: After myriad: Genetic testing in the wake of recent Supreme Court decisions about gene patents. *Curr Genet Med Rep 2*:223–241, 2014.

47. *NIH Battles Over Patent on Breast Cancer Gene.* The Washington Post, 1994.
48. Unit UsIP: Association for Molecular Pathology et al. v. Myriad Genetics, Inc. et al., 569 U.S. 12–398, 2013.
49. Walsh T, Lee MK, Casadei S, et al: Detection of inherited mutations for breast and ovarian cancer using genomic capture and massively parallel sequencing. *Proc Natl Acad Sci U S A 107*:12629–33, 2010.
50. Kolata G: Breaking ranks, lab offers test to assess risk of breast cancer. *N Y Times Web* A1, A15, 1996.
51. Cho MK, Sankar P, Wolpe PR, et al: Commercialization of BRCA1/2 testing: Practitioner awareness and use of a new genetic test. *Am J Med Genet 83*:157–63, 1999.
52. Holtzman NA, Murphy PD, Watson MS, et al: Predictive genetic testing: From basic research to clinical practice. *Science 278*:602–5, 1997.
53. Hubbard R, Lewontin RC: Pitfalls of genetic testing. *N Engl J Med 334*:1192–4, 1996.
54. Lawrence WF, Peshkin BN, Liang W, et al: Cost of genetic counseling and testing for BRCA1 and BRCA2 breast cancer susceptibility mutations. *Cancer Epidemiol Biomarkers Prev 10*:475–81, 2001.
55. Sturdy S: Framing utility: Regulatory reform and genetic tests in the USA, 1989–2000. *Soc Sci Med 304*:112924, 2022.
56. Smith O: Genetic testing: Out of the bottle. *Nature Medicine 2*:613–4, 1996.
57. Koenig B: Gene tests: What you know can hurt you. *New York Times*, 1996, pp 23.
58. Healy B: BRCA genes--bookmaking, fortunetelling, and medical care. *N Engl J Med 336*:1448–9, 1997.
59. Burke W, Kahn MJ, Garber JE, et al: "First do no harm" also applies to cancer susceptibility testing. *Cancer J Sci Am 2*:250–2, 1996.
60. Statement of the American Society of Clinical Oncology: genetic testing for cancer susceptibility, Adopted on February 20, 1996. *J Clin Oncol 14*:1730–6; discussion 1737–40, 1996.
61. Resource document for curriculum development in cancer genetics education. American Society of Clinical Oncology. *J Clin Oncol 15*:2157–69, 1997.
62. Holtzman N. A. WMS: Promoting Safe and Effective Genetic Testing in the United States: Final Report of the Task Force on Genetic Testing, 1997.
63. Levy-Lahad E, Catane R, Eisenberg S, et al: Founder BRCA1 and BRCA2 mutations in Ashkenazi Jews in Israel: frequency and differential penetrance in ovarian cancer and in breast-ovarian cancer families. *Am J Hum Genet 60*:1059–67, 1997.
64. Judkins T, Rosenthal E, Arnell C, et al: Clinical significance of large rearrangements in BRCA1 and BRCA2. *Cancer 118*:5210–6, 2012.
65. Matloff ET, Brierley KL: The double-helix derailed: the story of the BRCA patent. *Lancet 376*:314–5, 2010.
66. Daly MB, Axilbund JE, Buys SS, et al: Genetic/familial high-risk assessment: breast and ovarian, version 1.2013. *J Natl Compr Canc Netw, 8*:562–94, 2013
67. Laboratories MG: Integrated BRAC analysis to include BART, 2012.
68. Information NCfB: ClinVar.
69. BRCA Exchange.

70. Hudson KL: Prohibiting genetic discrimination. *N Engl J Med 356*:2021–3, 2007.

71. Hudson KL, Rothenberg KH, Andrews LB, et al: Genetic discrimination and health insurance: An urgent need for reform. *Science 270*:391–3, 1995.

72. Rothenberg K, Fuller B, Rothstein M, et al: Genetic information and the workplace: legislative approaches and policy changes. *Science 275*:1755–7, 1997.

73. Hudson KL, Holohan MK, Collins FS: Keeping pace with the times--the Genetic Information Nondiscrimination Act of 2008. *N Engl J Med 358*:2661–3, 2008.

74. Forrest IS, Chaudhary K, Vy HMT, et al: Population-based penetrance of deleterious clinical variants. *JAMA 327*:350–9, 2022.

75. Jackson L.W.M.N., Green HD, Mallabar-Rimmer B, Harrison JW, Wood AR, Ruth KS, Tyrrell J, Wright CF: *Influence of family history on penetrance of hereditary cancers in a population setting.* eClinicalMedicine, 2023.

76. Barnes DR, Rookus MA, McGuffog L, et al: Polygenic risk scores and breast and epithelial ovarian cancer risks for carriers of BRCA1 and BRCA2 pathogenic variants. *Genet Med 22*:1653–66, 2020.

77. Gupta S.W.J.M., Axell L, Burke CA, Chen L, Chung DC, Clayback KM, Dallas S, Felder S, Giardiello FM, Grady W, Hagemann A, Hall MJ, Hampel H, Hodan R, Idos G, Kassem N, Katona B, Lamps L, Llor X, Lu K, Markowitz AJ, Niell-Swiller M, Outlaw D, Pirzadeh-Miller S, Samadder NJ, Shibata D, Stanich PP, Swanson BJ, Szymaniak BM, Welborn J, Wiesner GL, Wolf A, Yurgelun MB: *National Comprehensive Cancer Network Guidelines Version 1.2023.* Genetic/ Familial High-Risk Assessment; Colorectal., 2023.

78. Meindl A, Hellebrand H, Wiek C, et al: Germline mutations in breast and ovarian cancer pedigrees establish RAD51C as a human cancer susceptibility gene. *Nat Genet 42*:410–4, 2010.

79. Yang X, Song H, Leslie G, et al: Ovarian and breast cancer risks associated with pathogenic variants in RAD51C and RAD51D. *J Natl Cancer Inst 112*:1242–50, 2020.

80. Loveday C, Turnbull C, Ramsay E, et al: Germline mutations in RAD51D confer susceptibility to ovarian cancer. *Nat Genet 43*:879–82, 2011.

81. Ramus SJ, Song H, Dicks E, et al: Germline mutations in the BRIP1, BARD1, PALB2, and NBN genes in women with ovarian cancer. *J Natl Cancer Inst 107*: 1–8, 2015.

82. Suszynska M, Ratajska M, Kozlowski P: BRIP1, RAD51C, and RAD51D mutations are associated with high susceptibility to ovarian cancer: Mutation prevalence and precise risk estimates based on a pooled analysis of ~30,000 cases. *J Ovarian Res 13*:50, 2020.

83. Weber-Lassalle N, Hauke J, Ramser J, et al: BRIP1 loss-of-function mutations confer high risk for familial ovarian cancer, but not familial breast cancer. *Breast Cancer Res 20*:7, 2018.

84. Rafnar T, Gudbjartsson DF, Sulem P, et al: Mutations in BRIP1 confer high risk of ovarian cancer. *Nat Genet 43*:1104–7, 2011.

85. Hall MJ, Bernhisel R, Hughes E, et al: Germline pathogenic variants in the ataxia telangiectasia mutated (ATM) gene are associated with high and moderate risks for multiple cancers. *Cancer Prev Res (Phila) 14*:433–40, 2021.

86. Kurian AW, Hughes E, Handorf EA, et al: Breast and ovarian cancer penetrance estimates derived from germline multiple-gene sequencing results in women. *JCO Precis Oncol 1*:1–12, 2017.

87. Narayan P, Ahsan MD, Webster EM, et al: Partner and localizer of BRCA2 (PALB2) pathogenic variants and ovarian cancer: A systematic review and meta-analysis. *Gynecol Oncol 177*:72–85, 2023.

88. Xia B, Sheng Q, Nakanishi K, et al: Control of BRCA2 cellular and clinical functions by a nuclear partner, PALB2. *Mol Cell 22*:719–29, 2006.

89. Yang X, Leslie G, Doroszuk A, et al: Cancer risks associated with germline PALB2 pathogenic variants: An international study of 524 families. *J Clin Oncol 38*:674–85, 2020.

90. Collaborative Group on Epidemiological Studies of Ovarian C, Beral V, Doll R, et al: Ovarian cancer and oral contraceptives: collaborative reanalysis of data from 45 epidemiological studies including 23,257 women with ovarian cancer and 87,303 controls. *Lancet 371*:303–14, 2008.

91. La Vecchia C: Oral contraceptives and ovarian cancer: an update, 1998–2004. *Eur J Cancer Prev 15*:117–24, 2006.

92. Baranska A, Kanadys W: Oral contraceptive use and breast cancer risk for BRCA1 and BRCA2 mutation carriers: Systematic review and meta-analysis of case-control studies. *Cancers (Basel) 14*:1–13, 2022.

93. van Bommel MHD, IntHout J, Veldmate G, et al: Contraceptives and cancer risks in BRCA1/2 pathogenic variant carriers: a systematic review and meta-analysis. *Hum Reprod Update 29*:197–217, 2023.

94. Labidi-Galy SI, Papp E, Hallberg D, et al: High grade serous ovarian carcinomas originate in the fallopian tube. *Nat Commun 8*:1093, 2017.

95. Steenbeek MP, van Bommel MHD, Inthout J, et al: TUBectomy with delayed oophorectomy as an alternative to risk-reducing salpingo-oophorectomy in high-risk women to assess the safety of prevention: the TUBA-WISP II study protocol. *Int J Gynecol Cancer 33*:982–7, 2023.

96. Domchek SM, Friebel TM, Singer CF, et al: Association of risk-reducing surgery in BRCA1 or BRCA2 mutation carriers with cancer risk and mortality. *JAMA 304*:967–75, 2010.

97. Finch AP, Lubinski J, Moller P, et al: Impact of oophorectomy on cancer incidence and mortality in women with a BRCA1 or BRCA2 mutation. *J Clin Oncol 32*:1547–53, 2014.

98. Kauff ND, Satagopan JM, Robson ME, et al: Risk-reducing salpingo-oophorectomy in women with a BRCA1 or BRCA2 mutation. *N Engl J Med 346*:1609–15, 2002.

99. Audeh MW, Carmichael J, Penson RT, et al: Oral poly(ADP-ribose) polymerase inhibitor olaparib in patients with BRCA1 or BRCA2 mutations and recurrent ovarian cancer: a proof-of-concept trial. *Lancet 376*:245–51, 2010.

100. Fong PC, Boss DS, Yap TA, et al: Inhibition of poly(ADP-ribose) polymerase in tumors from BRCA mutation carriers. *N Engl J Med 361*:123–34, 2009.

101. Fong PC, Yap TA, Boss DS, et al: Poly(ADP)-ribose polymerase inhibition: frequent durable responses in BRCA carrier ovarian cancer correlating with platinum-free interval. *J Clin Oncol 28*:2512–9, 2010.

102. Kaufman B, Shapira-Frommer R, Schmutzler RK, et al: Olaparib monotherapy in patients with advanced cancer and a germline BRCA1/2 mutation. *J Clin Oncol* 33:244–50, 2015.
103. Kim G, Ison G, McKee AE, et al: FDA approval summary: Olaparib monotherapy in patients with deleterious germline BRCA-mutated advanced ovarian cancer treated with three or more lines of chemotherapy. *Clin Cancer Res* 21:4257–61, 2015.
104. O'Malley DM, Krivak TC, Kabil N, et al: PARP inhibitors in ovarian cancer: A review. *Target Oncol* 18:471–503, 2023.
105. Moore K, Colombo N, Scambia G, et al: Maintenance olaparib in patients with newly diagnosed advanced ovarian cancer. *N Engl J Med* 379:2495–505, 2018.

History of PARP Inhibitors

4

Malte Renz and Jonathan S. Berek

4.1 INTRODUCTION

In this essay, we outline preclinical and clinical developments in PARP inhibitor use: from the discovery of the PARP enzyme in 1963 to the first FDA approval of PARP inhibitors in 2014 to the recent voluntary withdrawal of PARP inhibitors from late-line treatments of ovarian cancer and restrictions in second-line maintenance in 2022 and 2023, respectively. Figure 4.1 provides an abbreviated timeline of events. To focus on their history, we will omit here

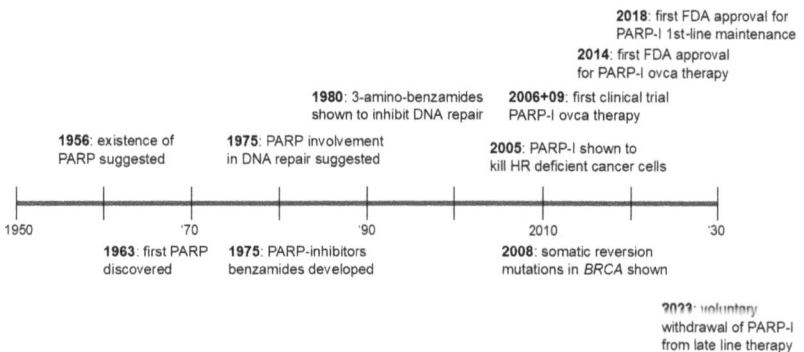

FIGURE 4.1 Timeline of the discovery, development, and clinical use of PARP inhibitors.

DOI: 10.1201/9781003312475-4

PARP-inhibitor mechanisms of action and resistance, since those are beyond the scope of this chapter and have been addressed elsewhere [1]. We hope that this historical outline of PARP-inhibitor development and use in ovarian cancer will provide context and understanding, including an indication of the temporary nature of medical knowledge.

4.2 CONCEPT

In contrast to other targeted therapies, which require the overactivity of a signaling cascade or the overexpression of a plasma membrane surface marker, the anti-cancer effect of PARP inhibitors depends upon an additional DNA damage repair defect in the targeted cancer cell, which renders the approach specific and spares normal cells. Synthetic lethality describes the requirement of two independent and complementary genetic hits that are tolerated individually but result in cell death if occurring together. This concept was originally applied to the model organism of the fruit fly, *Drosophila*, by Calvin Bridges in 1922 [2]. In 1946, Theodore Dobzhansky coined the actual term "synthetic lethality" [3]. According to the concept of synthetic lethality [2, 3], PARP inhibitors exploit a DNA repair deficiency of certain cancers (the first hit in the form of homologous repair deficiency) and overwhelm cancer cells with DNA aberrations (the second hit induced by PARP inhibitors) such that those cancer cells cannot repair, while normal cells harbor relevant intact DNA repair systems [4]. While other targeted therapies aim at protein kinases or surface membrane markers that are overexpressed and/or overactive and accelerate tumor growth and progression, the inhibition of PARP enzymes is the first example of targeting a non-essential DNA repair protein alone to treat cancer.

4.3 DISCOVERY AND DEVELOPMENT OF PARP INHIBITORS

In 1956, the existence of a cellular (poly) adenosine diphosphate (ADP)-ribose polymerase (PARP) was suggested by the profound depletion of NAD+ (nicotinamide adenine dinucleotide, at the time called DPN, which is diphosphopyridine nucleotide) during the exposure of cells to ethyleneimine, which is toxicologically similar to nitrogen mustard, alkylates DNA and thereby results in DNA damage. *Nicotinamide* appeared to inhibit this process [5]. Initially, these findings were interpreted as metabolic changes rather than DNA–damage related.

The first PARP enzyme was discovered and characterized by Paul Mandel's group in 1963. The group also described the enzyme product which they assumed to be polyadenylic acids [6]. The disappearance of NAD+ and simultaneous appearance of adenosine ribose polymers and *nicotinamide* was described in 1967 by Nishizuka et al. in a series of experiments [7]. In 1971, Preiss et al. [8] and Clark et al. [9] found that *nicotinamide* inhibits the PARP enzyme, likely by a negative feedback mechanism. In 1975, Edward Miller suggested the involvement of PARP enzymes in DNA repair [10]. In the same year, Sydney Shall's group described improved PARP inhibitors, the *benzamides*, close chemical analogues of *nicotinamide* [11]. *Benzamides* cannot be metabolized by NAD-biosynthetic enzymes because they lack the ring nitrogen of *nicotinamide*, which is their major advantage over other analogues of *nicotinamide*. Further development of *benzamides* resulted in the *3-aminobenzamides* [12] which are still being used as PARP inhibitors today. In the same year 1980, the Shall lab showed that *3-amino-benzamides* prevented DNA repair following exposure to the DNA methylating agent *dimethyl sulphate* [13].

Before a therapeutic role of PARP inhibitors in homologous recombination-deficient cancers was suspected, PARP inhibitors were developed as chemosensitizers and radiosensitizers. The PARP inhibitor AG14361, a forerunner to *rucaparib*, was reported to enhance the antiproliferative activity of *temozolomide*, an alkylating agent; *topotecan*, a topoisomerase 1 inhibitor; and to inhibit the recovery of cancer cells from gamma irradiation [14]. In 2005, the first reported phase I trial tested the PARP inhibitor AG14699 and *temozolomide* in solid cancers [15].

In the same year, two groups showed that the inhibition of a non-essential DNA repair system can be used to kill cancer cells that lack homologous recombination (HR), a DNA double strand repair mechanism [16, 17]. Their work has been published back-to-back by Bryant et al. and Farmer et al. [16, 17]. The inhibition of PARP results in single strand breaks that degenerate into double strand breaks and eventually result in the collapse of DNA replication. Unrepaired double strand breaks in HR–deficient cells lead to cell death. HR–deficient cells include BRCA–mutated cells and cells with deficiencies in other genes that are involved in the complex homologous repair mechanism [18]. Bryant et al. used for their experiments NU1025 and AG14361, forerunners to *rucaparib*. Farmer et al. used KU0058684 and KU0058948, forerunners to *olaparib*.

Shortly after this seminal work, in 2008, *BRCA1/2* reversion mutations were reported in pancreatic cancer and ovarian cancer cell lines [19, 20].

Secondary mutations were found to restore the *BRCA1/2* open reading frame. These secondary mutations were more frequently detected in ovarian cancers, which had been exposed to multiple chemotherapies, especially platinum-resistant epithelial ovarian cancers. Most secondary *BRCA1* or *2* mutations take place after platinum chemotherapy. In autopsy studies, many distinct reversion events in the same patient have been identified, contributing to the intra-patient heterogeneity of ovarian cancer [21]. Over the years, several PARP-inhibitor resistance mechanisms have been described, which we lay out elsewhere [1].

4.4 INITIAL CLINICAL TRIALS AND FDA APPROVAL

Preclinical data showed that *BRCA1*- and *BRCA2*-deficient cells were up to 1000-fold more sensitive to PARP inhibition than wild-type cells. Tumor growth was inhibited in *BRCA2*-deficient xenografts [16, 17, 22] and genetically engineered *BRCA1*-associated breast cancer mouse models [23].

Preliminary results of the first single-agent *olaparib* (AZD2281) phase I trial were initially presented on patients unselected for BRCA mutation [24]. Given the preclinical data published in 2005, this trial then focused on germline BRCA–mutated patients [25]. Of the 60 patients enrolled, 22 were carriers of *BRCA1* or *BRCA2* mutation. After dose escalation another cohort was enrolled comprising only *BRCA* mutation carriers that received 200 mg *olaparib* twice daily. Objective responses were reported only in mutation carriers, all of whom had ovarian, breast, or prostate cancer and had received multiple treatments. Results of a phase II trial of single agent *olaparib* in recurrent germline BRCA–mutated ovarian cancer were published in 2009/2010 [26, 27]. This multicenter trial enrolled two cohorts of 33 and 24 patients with recurrent ovarian cancer with germline *BRCA1* and *BRCA2* mutations, who received 400 mg twice daily and 100 mg twice daily. The objective response rate was 33% and 13% in the 400 mg and 100 mg cohorts, respectively. The trial data was published back to back with the data on recurrent breast cancer; the objective response rates here were 41% and 22%, respectively [28].

Kaufman et al. reported study results of *olaparib* monotherapy in patients with germline *BRCA* mutations and advanced *BRCA*–associated cancers, including ovarian cancer, that were platinum resistant or unsuitable for further platinum therapy. An objective response rate of 26% was noted across tumor types and 31% in ovarian cancer patients [29]. This study combined with results of study 19 (see next paragraph) lead to FDA approval of *olaparib* in December 2014 as the first monotherapy for patients with deleterious or suspected deleterious germline *BRCA*–mutated advanced ovarian cancer who have been treated with three or more prior lines of chemotherapy [30].

Study 19 addressed late-line maintenance therapy in recurrent platinum-sensitive ovarian cancer. First results regardless of *BRCA* status were published in 2012 [31]. In 2014, a preplanned retrospective analysis of the trial outcomes by *BRCA* status and matured overall survival data were published [32] and supported greatest benefit with a *BRCA* mutation. Final overall survival analysis published in 2016 showed an improvement of 34.9 versus 30.2 months with a *BRCA* mutation and 24.6 months versus 26.6 months without a *BRCA* mutation [33].

An early trial on late line treatment, i.e., ≥ 3 lines, in patients with a germline *BRCA* mutation regardless of platinum-sensitivity was Study 42 [34]. The objective response rate overall in 193 patients was 34% and in patients with platinum-resistant disease 30% with a median duration of response of 8.0 months. In the sequel, PARP inhibitor use was moved up from late-line treatment to upfront first-line maintenance therapy. The current use is outlined next.

4.5 CURRENT USE

Over the years, increasing evidence has accumulated to support the role of maintenance therapy with PARP inhibitors following response to treatment in the first-line therapy setting as well as in patients with platinum-sensitive recurrent ovarian cancer.

4.6 FIRST-LINE SINGLE-AGENT MAINTENANCE THERAPY

Olaparib: In the SOLO1 trial, patients with Stage III and IV high-grade serous/high-grade endometrioid ovarian cancer, a germline or somatic *BRCA1* or 2 mutation, and at least partial response to adjuvant platinum-based chemotherapy were randomized to *olaparib* maintenance or placebo [35]. A 70% risk reduction for progression of disease or death was seen for *olaparib* (HR 0.3) with a median progression-free survival not reached versus 13.8 months with placebo. Twice as many patients were progression free after 3 years (60.4% vs. 26.9%), which is unprecedented. At 5-year follow-up, 48% of patients randomized to 2 years of *olaparib* were progression free compared with 21% in the placebo arm. The median progression-free survival was 56 months versus 13.8 months (HR 0.33) [36]. At the 7-year follow-up, 45.3% of *olaparib* patients versus 20.6% of the placebo patients were alive and had not received the first subsequent treatment. The hazard ratio for overall survival was 0.55 (95% CI, 0.4–0.76; p = 0.0004 [p < 0.0001 was required to declare statistical significance]) [37].

Niraparib: The PRIMA trial enrolled a subset of patients considered to be at high risk of relapse and included patients with Stage III and IV high-grade serous and endometrioid ovarian cancer with response to chemotherapy, regardless of *BRCA* status. The trial included those with suboptimal residual disease for Stage III after surgery as well as patients who received NACT and all patients with Stage IV [38]. Patients were randomized to niraparib or placebo for 3 years. In the overall population, the median progression-free survival was 8.2 months versus 13.8 months (control vs. niraparib). In the homologous recombination deficient (HRD) subgroup as determined by the Myriad myChoice test (Myriad Genetics Inc, Salt Lake City, USA), the median progression-free survival was 10.9 months versus 22.1 months. In the homologous recombination proficient subgroup, the difference was smaller, although statistically significant (5.4 months vs. 8.1 months). Final overall survival results after a median follow-up of 73.9 months showed no difference in the treatment arms in the overall, HRD and HRP population [39].

The PRIME trial which evaluated niraparib as first-line maintenance in 384 Chinese patients with newly diagnosed advanced ovarian cancer showed similar results. The median PFS improved in the intention to treat population compared to placebo (24.8 months vs. 8.3 months) and in the studied subgroups. Median PFS was not reached versus 10.8 months in patients with germline *BRCA* mutation and 19.3 versus 8.3 months in patients without germline *BRCA* mutation; not reached versus 11 months in HRD patients and 16.6 versus 5.5 in HRP patients [40].

In both trials, *niraparib* dosing was reduced to 200 mg if the body weight was less than 77 kg and platelet count less than 150 $10^3/\mu l$ [41].

Rucaparib: The ATHENA-MONO trial studied *rucaparib* as first-line maintenance. Median PFS was 28.7 months versus 11.3 months for the HRD patients (*rucaparib* vs. placebo) and 12.1 months versus 9.1 months in the HRD–negative (or HRP) patients which was maintained at the 4-year follow-up [42, 43].

4.7 FIRST-LINE MAINTENANCE COMBINATION THERAPY

4.7.1 Rationale for Combining PARP Inhibitors with VEGF Inhibitors

The VEGF (vascular endothelial growth factor) pathway has been shown to modify the homologous recombination DNA repair system. For example, inhibition of VEGFR-3 results in downregulation of *BRCA1* and *BRCA2* gene expression [44]; angiogenesis inhibition by VEGF inhibitors induces hypoxia, which in turn downregulates *RAD51* [45]. Thereby, angiogenesis inhibitors induce a homologous deficient state and render cancer cells sensitive to PARP inhibition.

Olaparib + bevacizumab: In the PAOLA-1 trial, patients with Stage III–IV high-grade serous cancers, regardless of BRCA status and at least partial response, were randomized to *bevacizumab* or *bevacizumab* plus *olaparib* maintenance therapy [46]. The median progression-free survival for the intention-to-treat population was 16.6 months versus 22.1 months (without versus with olaparib). In the *BRCA*–mutated group, median progression-free survival was 21.7 months versus 37.2 months and in the HRD group excluding *BRCA*, median progression-free survival was 16.6 months versus 28.1 months. However, in the HRD–negative or unknown group the median progression-free survival showed no difference (16 months vs. 16.9 months). The PAOLA design did not include *olaparib* monotherapy, making it difficult to ascertain the contribution of bevacizumab. Nevertheless, the *olaparib* plus *bevacizumab* combination received FDA approval as first-line maintenance for HRD patients.

Data from another first-line combination maintenance trial, DUO-O, was recently presented [47]. The three-arm phase III trial randomized patients with advanced ovarian cancer without somatic or germline *BRCA* mutation but stratified by HRD/ HRP. Patients in arm 1 received *carboplatin/ paclitaxel* plus *bevacizumab* followed by *bevacizumab* maintenance, in arm 2 *carboplatin/ paclitaxel* plus *durvalumab* plus *bevacizumab* followed by *durvalumab* plus *bevacizumab* maintenance, and in arm 3 *carboplatin/ paclitaxel* plus *durvalumab* plus *bevacizumab* followed by *durvalumab* plus *bevacizumab* plus *olaparib* maintenance. An improvement in medina PFS was seen between arm 3 and arm 1: in HRD patients 37.3

months versus 23.0 months (HR, 0.49; 95% CI, 0.34–0.69), in the intention to treat population 24.2 months versus 19.3 months (HR, 0.63; 95% CI, 0.52–0.76), and in the HRP or HRD–negative patients 20.9 months versus 17.4 months (HR, 0.69; 95% CI, 0.54–0.86).

4.8 RATIONALE FOR COMBINING PARP INHIBITORS WITH IMMUNE CHECKPOINT INHIBITORS

Increased DNA damage results in increased genomic instability, a higher mutational burden, and thereby an increased neoantigen release and presentation. For example, HR–deficient tumors have been shown to have higher numbers of CD3+ and CD8+ tumor-infiltrating lymphocytes (TILs) and increased PD-L1 expression [48]. PARP inhibitors have been shown to inactivate GSK3α/β (glycogen synthase kinase-3) and thereby increase PD-L1 expression [49].

Rucaparib + nivolumab and olaparib + durvalumab: Despite the strong theoretical rationale for combining immune checkpoint inhibitors with a PARP inhibitor, the ATHENA-COMBO trial investigating *nivolumab* and *rucaparib* versus *rucaparib* and *placebo* was a negative trial [50]. COMBO was associated with a numerically shorter mean PFS than MONO in the intention-to-treat population and HRD and PD-L1 subgroups. At data cut off 2 of the DUO-O trial, PFS benefit of arm 3 (*durvalumab + carboplatin + paclitaxel + bevacizumab* followed by *durvalumab + bevacizumab + Olaparib*) versus arm 1 (control: *carboplatin + paclitaxel + bevacizumab* followed by *bevacizumab*) was sustained in the non-*BRCAm* HRD and non-*BRCAm* ITT group [51], just as at the prior data cut off [47]. However, it is challenging to interpret the results of DUO-O because the combination of *olaparib* and *durvalumab* and *bevacizumab* was superior to the control of *bevacizumab* as well as the *bevacizumab* and *durvalumab* arm. Ideally, there should have been an arm with a PARP inhibitor with *bevacizumab*. Without that comparison, the contribution of immune checkpoint inhibitor to *olaparib* and *bevacizumab* cannot be determined. Further studies are required to determine the role for immune checkpoint inhibitors in the first-line treatment of patients with ovarian cancer or whether it is possible to identify a subset who are most likely to derive benefit.

4.9 SECOND-LINE OR GREATER SINGLE-AGENT MAINTENANCE THERAPY

PARP inhibitors, including *niraparib* and *olaparib*, have been approved by the FDA in the recurrent setting for 2nd line or greater maintenance therapy in patients with platinum-sensitive disease following a partial or complete response to platinum-based chemotherapy, initially regardless of *BRCA* status. The PFS is improved with these agents regardless of the *BRCA* status, although the patients with *BRCA* germline/somatic mutations have a greater benefit than patients without mutations. Long term follow-up of the overall survival showed a potential detriment for patients without a *BRCA* mutation. In the fall 2023, the FDA restricted the *niraparib* and *olaparib* second-line maintenance indications to patients with *BRCA* germline or *BRCA* germline and somatic mutations, respectively.

Niraparib has been approved by the U.S. FDA for second-line or greater maintenance therapy in patients with platinum-sensitive disease following a partial or complete response to platinum-based chemotherapy for germline *BRCA1* and *BRCA2* carriers.

In the NOVA study, a phase III trial, 553 patients with platinum-sensitive recurrent ovarian cancer were assigned randomly after completion of platinum-based chemotherapy in a 2:1 ratio to *niraparib* maintenance or placebo. Patients were stratified based on the presence or absence of a *gBRCA* mutation. The patients in the non–*gBRCA* mutation cohort were further classified by whether HRD was observed. *Niraparib* compared to placebo increased the PFS in all groups of patients. In the *gBRCA* group, the PFS was 21 months versus 5.5 months (HR, 0.27; 95% CI, 0.17–0.41) in contrast to the non–*gBRCA* group, where the PFS was 9.3 months versus 3.9 months (HR, 0.45; 95% CI, 0.34–0.61). This study also attempted to identify the subset of patients with tumors with HRD and reported that in the HRD–positive group of non–*gBRCA* patients, the PFS was 12.9 months versus 3.8 months (HR, 0.38; 95% CI, 0.24–0.59). An exploratory analysis of HRD–negative patients demonstrated an improvement in the median PFS in favor of *niraparib* (6.9 months vs. 3.8 months; HR, 0.58; 95% CI, 0.08–0.90) [52]. Long-term follow-up showed a potential, statistically non-significant detriment to the overall survival of the non–*gBRCA* patients (31.1 months vs. 36.5 months; HR, 1.1; 95% CI, 0.83–1.46) and the non–*gBRCA*, but HRD-positive patients (37.3 months vs. 41.1 months; HR, 1.32; 95% CI, 0.84–2.06). This data resulted in 'Dear Health Care Provider' Letters by the pharmaceutical industry in May 2022 [53]. In an updated OS (overall survival) analysis accounting for missing survival data a similar trend was seen and resulted in another Healthcare Provider Letter in November 2022 [54] and the FDA restriction of the niraparib approval to second-line maintenance for *gBRCA* patients only. In March 2023, further long-term data was presented and confirmed no statistically significant difference in overall survival in any of the pre-defined subgroups [55]. It has been pointed out that the study was not powered to derive overall or subgroup survival information.

Olaparib is FDA approved for the second-line or greater maintenance therapy of patients with a germline or somatic *BRCA* mutation and platinum-sensitive recurrent ovarian cancer and complete or partial response.

There are data in support of maintenance *olaparib* in women with platinum-sensitive recurrent high-grade serous ovarian cancer from Study 19. This was a randomized phase II controlled trial of approximately 300 women with platinum-sensitive recurrent high-grade ovarian cancer who had achieved a response to their most recent treatment regardless of their BRCA status. The patients were randomly assigned to *olaparib* 400 mg twice daily or placebo. Compared with placebo, *olaparib* was shown to improve the PFS (8 months vs. 5 months; HR for progression or death, 0.35; 95% CI, 0.25–0.49) [31]. A separate analysis of Study 19 evaluated outcomes for *gBRCA* patients and showed that the clinical benefit was greatest for these patients. The PFS was (11 months vs. 4 months; HR, 0.18; 95% CI, 0.10–0.31) for *olaparib* versus placebo, respectively [32, 33].

These results were confirmed in the much larger SOLO2 trial, which included 295 patients with *gBRCA* mutations and platinum-sensitive recurrent ovarian cancer who had responded to platinum-based chemotherapy. They were randomly assigned to receive *olaparib* ($n = 196$) or placebo ($n = 99$). The median PFS was significantly longer with *olaparib* (19.1 months [95% CI, 16.3–25.7]) compared to placebo (5.5 months [5.2–5.8]; HR, 0.30; 95% CI, 0.22–0.41]; $p < 0.0001$) [56].

The decision to restrict the second-line maintenance treatment to *BRCA*–mutated patients (germline or somatic mutations) was based on randomized trials with other PARP inhibitors and was communicated in a Healthcare Provider Letter in September 2023 [57].

Rucaparib is approved for second-line maintenance therapy of *BRCA*-mutation–associated advanced ovarian cancer after completion of treatment with two or more chemotherapy regimens with partial or complete response.

Ariel 3 included patients with platinum-sensitive, high-grade serous or endometrioid ovarian, fallopian tube, or peritoneal carcinoma, who had received at least two prior platinum-based chemotherapy regimens, complete or partial response to their last platinum-based regimen, and a CA-125 concentration of less than the upper limit of normal. They were randomized 2:1 to receive oral *rucaparib* 600 mg twice daily or placebo. The median PFS in patients with a BRCA–mutant carcinoma was 16.6 months (95% CI, 13.4–22.9; 130 [35%] patients) in the *rucaparib* group versus 5.4 months (3.4–6.7; 66 [35%] patients) in the placebo group (HR, 0.23 [95% CI, 0.16–0.34]; $p < 0.0001$). Similar to the NOVA trial, the investigators analyzed all tumors for HRD using a different method. In patients with an HRD carcinoma (236 [63%] in the *rucaparib* group versus 118 [62%] in the placebo group), the PFS was 13.6 months (10.9–16.2) versus 5.4 months (5.1–5.6; HR 0.32 [95% CI 0.24–0.42]; $p < 0.0001$) [58]. Long-term follow-up of overall survival was recently presented [59] and showed a similar trend to the NOVA trial for niraparib. While the PFS showed a statistically significant difference for *BRCA*–mutated (26.1 months vs. 18.4 months, p = 0.02) and HRD-positive patients (24.7 months vs. 18.4 months; p = 0.01), the overall survival showed no statistically significant difference (*BRCA* patients: 45.9 months vs. 47.8 months; 95% CI, 0.58–1.19; p = 0.32) with a trend in the HRD patients to a potential survival detriment (40.5 months vs. 47.8 months; 95% CI, 0.77–1.32; p = 0.97). Like the NOVA trial, Ariel 3 was not powered to evaluate between-groups OS differences. This data resulted in the FDA restriction of the approval to *BRCA*–mutation associated advanced ovarian cancers.

4.10 LATE-LINE TREATMENT AND VOLUNTARY WITHDRAWAL

The initial approval of PARP inhibitors for late-line treatment was based on the following studies: study 42 for *olaparib* [34], the QUADRA study for *niraparib [60]*, and an integrated analysis of data from study 10 part 2A and Ariel 2 parts 1 and 2 for *rucaparib* [61]. At the final overall survival analysis of the Ariel 4 trial, a possible detriment in OS was seen for *rucaparib* (median OS 19.4 months vs. 25.4 months in the ITT population, and 14.2 months vs. 22.2 months in the platinum resistant group) [62]. Furthermore, a post-hoc analysis of SOLO3 found a potential detriment for *olaparib* in patients who had received three or more prior lines [63]. Neither Ariel 4 nor SOLO3 were powered to assess between-group differences in OS. These trial results lead to 'Dear Health Care Provider Letters' in June and August 2022 for *rucaparib* and *olaparib*. Based on the totality of data and the single-arm nature of the QUADRA trial which prevents the assessment of OS data, a letter for *niraparib* followed in September 2022. Subsequently, these PARP inhibitors were voluntarily withdrawn by the pharmaceutical companies for the single-agent PARP inhibitor treatment in late line [64]. The final overall survival results of the SOLO3 trial showed a possible detrimental effect for patients who had received at least three previous chemotherapy lines (HR 1.33, 95% CI, 0.84–2.18; median 29.9 vs. 39.4 months) [65].

4.11 CONCLUSION

PARP inhibitors are the first example of exploiting a DNA repair deficiency in cancer cells by targeting non-essential DNA repair systems and thus inducing synthetic lethality only in cancer cells with the underlying DNA repair defect. The first FDA approval was granted in 2014 for the late-line treatment in heavily pretreated recurrent ovarian cancer; an application that was eventually voluntarily withdrawn in 2023. Although the evidence for the withdrawal appears sparse, the impact of PARP inhibitors in first- and second-line maintenance seems clear for cancers with germline and somatic *BRCA* mutations and defects in homologous repair as detected by the functional surrogate HRD testing. Further indications of PARP inhibitors include combinations with *bevacizumab* and possibly in the future with other targeted or immunotherapies.

REFERENCES

1. Renz M, Berek JS, Dorigo O, Biologic, targeted, and immune therapy. in Berek J, Hacker N, eds, *Berek and Hacker's Gynecologic Oncology*, Lippincott Williams & Wilkins (LWW). 2020: 36–59.
2. Bridges CB, The origin of variations in sexual and sex-limited characters. *The American Naturalist*, 1922;**56**:51–63.
3. Dobzhansky T, Genetics of natural populations; recombination and variability in populations of Drosophila pseudoobscura. *Genetics*, 1946;**31**:269–90.
4. Brody LC, Treating cancer by targeting a weakness. *N Engl J Med*, 2005; **353**(9):949–50.
5. Roitt IM, The inhibition of carbohydrate metabolism in ascites-tumour cells by ethyleneimines. *Biochem J*, 1956;**63**(2):300–7.
6. Chambon P, Weill JD, Mandel P, Nicotinamide mononucleotide activation of new DNA-dependent polyadenylic acid synthesizing nuclear enzyme. *Biochem Biophys Res Commun*, 1963;**11**:39–43.
7. Nishizuka Y et al., Studies on the polymer of adenosine diphosphate ribose. I. Enzymic formation from nicotinamide adenine dinuclotide in mammalian nuclei. *J Biol Chem*, 1967;**242**(13):3164–71.
8. Preiss J, Schlaeger R, Hilz R, Specific inhibition of poly adpribose polymerase by thymidine and nicotinamide in HeLa cells. *FEBS Lett*, 1971;**19**(3):244–6.

9. Clark JB, Ferris GM, Pinder S, Inhibition of nuclear NAD nucleosidase and poly ADP-ribose polymerase activity from rat liver by nicotinamide and 5'-methyl nicotinamide. *Biochim Biophys Acta*, 1971;**238**(1):82–5.

10. Miller EG, Stimulation of nuclear poly (adenosine diphosphate-ribose) polymerase activity from HeLa cells by endonucleases. *Biochim Biophys Acta*, 1975;**395**(2):191–200.

11. Shall, S., Proceedings: Experimental manipulation of the specific activity of poly(ADP-ribose) polymerase. *J Biochem*, 1975;**77**(1):2.

12. Purnell MR, Whish WJ, Novel inhibitors of poly(ADP-ribose) synthetase. *Biochem J*, 1980;**185**(3):775–7.

13. Durkacz BW et al., *(ADP-ribose)n participates in DNA excision repair. Nature*, 1980;**283**(5747):593–6.

14. Calabrese CR et al., Anticancer chemosensitization and radiosensitization by the novel poly(ADP-ribose) polymerase-1 inhibitor AG14361. *J Natl Cancer Inst*, 2004;**96**(1):56–67.

15. Plummer R et al., First in human phase I trial of the PARP inhibitor AG-014699 with temozolomide (TMZ) in patients (pts) with advanced solid tumors. *Journal of Clinical Oncology*, 2005;**23**(16_suppl):3065.

16. Bryant HE et al., Specific killing of BRCA2-deficient tumours with inhibitors of poly(ADP-ribose) polymerase. *Nature*, 2005;**434**(7035):913–7.

17. Farmer H et al., Targeting the DNA repair defect in BRCA mutant cells as a therapeutic strategy. *Nature*, 2005;**434**(7035):917–21.

18. McCabe N et al., Deficiency in the repair of DNA damage by homologous recombination and sensitivity to poly(ADP-ribose) polymerase inhibition. *Cancer Res*, 2006;**66**(16):8109–15.

19. Edwards SL et al., Resistance to therapy caused by intragenic deletion in BRCA2. *Nature*, 2008;**451**(7182):1111–5.

20. Sakai W et al., Secondary mutations as a mechanism of cisplatin resistance in BRCA2-mutated cancers. *Nature*, 2008;**451**(7182):1116–20.

21. Patch AM et al., Whole-genome characterization of chemoresistant ovarian cancer. *Nature*, 2015;**521**(7553):489–94.

22. Evers B et al., Selective inhibition of BRCA2-deficient mammary tumor cell growth by AZD2281 and cisplatin. *Clin Cancer Res*, 2008;**14**(12):3916–25.

23. Rottenberg S et al., High sensitivity of BRCA1-deficient mammary tumors to the PARP inhibitor AZD2281 alone and in combination with platinum drugs. *Proc Natl Acad Sci USA*, 2008;**105**(44):17079–84.

24. Fong PC et al., Phase I pharmacokinetic (PK) and pharmacodynamic (PD) evaluation of a small molecule inhibitor of Poly ADP-Ribose Polymerase (PARP), KU-0059436 (Ku) in patients (p) with advanced tumours. *J Clin Oncol* 2006;**24**(18_suppl):3022.

25. Fong PC et al., Inhibition of poly(ADP-ribose) polymerase in tumors from BRCA mutation carriers. *N Engl J Med*, 2009;**361**(2):123–34.

26. Audeh MW et al., Phase II trial of the oral PARP inhibitor olaparib (AZD2281) in BRCA-deficient advanced ovarian cancer. *J Clin Oncol* 2009;**27**(15_suppl): 5500.

27. Audeh MW et al., Oral poly(ADP-ribose) polymerase inhibitor olaparib in patients with BRCA1 or BRCA2 mutations and recurrent ovarian cancer: a proof-of-concept trial. *Lancet*, 2010;**376**(9737):245–51.

28. Tutt A et al., Oral poly(ADP-ribose) polymerase inhibitor olaparib in patients with BRCA1 or BRCA2 mutations and advanced breast cancer: a proof-of-concept trial. *Lancet*, 2010;**376**(9737):235–44.
29. Kaufman B et al., Olaparib monotherapy in patients with advanced cancer and a germline BRCA1/2 mutation. *J Clin Oncol*, 2015;**33**(3):244–50.
30. AstraZeneca. *LYNPARZA™ approved by the US food and drug administration for the treatment of advanced ovarian cancer in patients with germline BRCA-mutations [internet]* 2014: www.astrazeneca.com/media-centre/press-releases/2014/lynparza-approved-us-fda-brca-mutated-ovarian-cancer-treatment-19122014.html#
31. Ledermann J et al., Olaparib maintenance therapy in platinum-sensitive relapsed ovarian cancer. *N Engl J Med*, 2012;**366**(15):1382–92.
32. Ledermann J et al., Olaparib maintenance therapy in patients with platinum-sensitive relapsed serous ovarian cancer: a preplanned retrospective analysis of outcomes by BRCA status in a randomised phase 2 trial. *Lancet Oncol*, 2014;**15**(8):852–61.
33. Ledermann JA et al., Overall survival in patients with platinum-sensitive recurrent serous ovarian cancer receiving olaparib maintenance monotherapy: an updated analysis from a randomised, placebo-controlled, double-blind, phase 2 trial. *Lancet Oncol*, 2016;**17**(11):1579–89.
34. Domchek SM et al., Efficacy and safety of olaparib monotherapy in germline BRCA1/2 mutation carriers with advanced ovarian cancer and three or more lines of prior therapy. *Gynecol Oncol*, 2016;**140**(2):199–203.
35. Moore K et al., Maintenance olaparib in patients with newly diagnosed advanced ovarian cancer. *N Engl J Med*, 2018;**379**(26):2495–505.
36. Banerjee S et al., Maintenance olaparib for patients with newly diagnosed advanced ovarian cancer and a BRCA mutation (SOLO1/GOG 3004): 5-year follow-up of a randomised, double-blind, placebo-controlled, phase 3 trial. *Lancet Oncol*, 2021;**22**(12):1721–31.
37. DiSilvestro P et al., Overall survival with maintenance olaparib at a 7-year follow-up in patients with newly diagnosed advanced ovarian cancer and a BRCA mutation: The SOLO1/GOG 3004 trial. *J Clin Oncol*, 2023;**41**(3):609–17.
38. Gonzalez-Martin A et al., Niraparib in Patients with Newly Diagnosed Advanced Ovarian Cancer. *N Engl J Med*, 2019;**381**(25):2391–402.
39. Monk BJ et al., Niraparib first-line maintenance therapy in patients with newly diagnosed advanced ovarian cancer: final overall survival results from the PRIMA/ENGOT-OV26/GOG-3012 trial☆. *Ann Oncol*, 2024;**35**(11):981–92.
40. Li N et al., Treatment with niraparib maintenance therapy in patients with newly diagnosed advanced ovarian cancer: A phase 3 randomized clinical trial. *JAMA Oncol*, 2023;**9**(9):1230–37.
41. Berek JS et al., Safety and dose modification for patients receiving niraparib. *Ann Oncol*, 2018;**29**(8):1784–92.
42. Monk BJ et al., A Randomized, Phase III Trial to Evaluate Rucaparib Monotherapy as Maintenance Treatment in Patients With Newly Diagnosed Ovarian Cancer (ATHENA-MONO/GOG-3020/ENGOT-ov45). *J Clin Oncol*, 2022;**40**(34):3952–64.
43. Kristeleit R et al., 49MO Updated progression-free survival (PFS) in patients (pts) with newly diagnosed advanced ovarian cancer (OC) treated with rucaparib (RUC) in ATHENA-MONO. *ESMO Open*, 2024;**9**:5.

44. Lim JJ et al., VEGFR3 inhibition chemosensitizes ovarian cancer stemlike cells through down-regulation of BRCA1 and BRCA2. *Neoplasia*, 2014;**16**(4):343–53.
45. Bindra RS et al., Down-regulation of Rad51 and decreased homologous recombination in hypoxic cancer cells. *Mol Cell Biol*, 2004;**24**(19):8504–18.
46. Ray-Coquard I et al., Olaparib plus bevacizumab as first-line maintenance in ovarian cancer. *N Engl J Med*, 2019;**381**(25):2416–28.
47. Harter P et al., Durvalumab with paclitaxel/carboplatin (PC) and bevacizumab (bev), followed by maintenance durvalumab, bev, and olaparib in patients (pts) with newly diagnosed advanced ovarian cancer (AOC) without a tumor BRCA1/2 mutation (non-tBRCAm): Results from the randomized, placebo (pbo)-controlled phase III DUO-O trial. *J Clin Oncol*, 2023;**41**(17_suppl):LBA5506–LBA5506.
48. Strickland KC et al., Association and prognostic significance of BRCA1/2-mutation status with neoantigen load, number of tumor-infiltrating lymphocytes and expression of PD-1/PD-L1 in high grade serous ovarian cancer. *Oncotarget*, 2016;**7**(12):13587–98.
49. Jiao S et al., PARP Inhibitor Upregulates PD-L1 Expression and Enhances Cancer-Associated Immunosuppression. *Clin Cancer Res*, 2017;**23**(14):3711–20.
50. Monk BJ et al., LBA30 ATHENA-COMBO, a phase III, randomized trial comparing rucaparib (RUCA) + nivolumab (NIVO) combination therapy vs RUCA monotherapy as maintenance treatment in patients (pts) with newly diagnosed ovarian cancer (OC). *Ann Oncol*, 2024;**35**:S1223–S1224.
51. Trillsch F et al., Durvalumab (D) + carboplatin/paclitaxel (CP) + bevacizumab (B) followed by D, B + olaparib (O) maintenance (mtx) for newly diagnosed advanced ovarian cancer (AOC) without a tumour BRCA1/BRCA2 mutation (non-tBRCAm): Updated results from DUO-O, *ESMO*. *Ann Oncol*. 2024;**9**:5103550.
52. Mirza MR et al., Niraparib Maintenance Therapy in Platinum-Sensitive, Recurrent Ovarian Cancer. *N Engl J Med*, 2016;**375**(22):2154–64.
53. GSK, *Dear Health Care Provider Letter (Niraparib)*, 2022.
54. GSK, *Dear Health Care Provider Letter*. 2022.
55. Matulonis UA, Herrstedt J, Oza A et al. Final overall survival and long-term safety in the ENGOT-OV16/NOVA phase III trial of niraparib in patients with recurrent ovarian cancer. In *Society of Gynecologic Oncology Annual Meeting on Women's Cancer*. 2023.
56. Pujade-Lauraine E et al., Olaparib tablets as maintenance therapy in patients with platinum-sensitive, relapsed ovarian cancer and a BRCA1/2 mutation (SOLO2/ENGOT-Ov21): a double-blind, randomised, placebo-controlled, phase 3 trial. *Lancet Oncol*, 2017;**18**(9):1274–84.
57. AstraZeneca. *Dear Health Care Provider*, 2023: www.lynparzahcp.com/content/dam/physician-services/us/590-lynparza-hcp-branded/hcp-global/pdf/solo3-dhcp-final-signed.pdf.
58. Coleman RL et al., Rucaparib maintenance treatment for recurrent ovarian carcinoma after response to platinum therapy (ARIEL3): a randomised, double-blind, placebo-controlled, phase 3 trial. *Lancet*, 2017;**390**(10106):1949–61.
59. Coleman RL et al., O003/#557 Overall survival results from ARIEL3: a phase 3 randomized, double-blind study of rucaparib vs placebo following response to platinum-based chemotherapy for recurrent ovarian carcinoma. *Int J Gynecol Cancer*, 2022;**32**(Suppl 3):A3–A4.

60. Moore KN et al., Niraparib monotherapy for late-line treatment of ovarian cancer (QUADRA): a multicentre, open-label, single-arm, phase 2 trial. *Lancet Oncol*, 2019;**20**(5):636–48.

61. Oza AM et al., Antitumor activity and safety of the PARP inhibitor rucaparib in patients with high-grade ovarian carcinoma and a germline or somatic BRCA1 or BRCA2 mutation: Integrated analysis of data from Study 10 and ARIEL2. *Gynecol Oncol*, 2017;**147**(2):267–75.

62. Oza AM, Lisyanskaya AS, Fedenko AA et al. *Overall survival results from ARIEL4: A phase III study assessing rucaparib vs chemotherapy in patients with advanced, relapsed ovarian carcinoma and a deleterious BRCA1/2 mutation.* ESMO. 2022.

63. Leath CA, Scambia G, Valencia RV et al. Overall survival by number of prior lines of chemotherapy in patients with BRCA-mutated platinum-sensitive relapsed ovarian cancer receiving olaparib treatment or non-platinum chemotherapy in SOLO3. In *IGCS Annual Global Meeting*. 2022. New York.

64. Society of Gynecologic Oncologists Clinical Practice. *Summary: Revisions to FDA approvals for PARP Inhibitors in the management of ovarian cancer.* 2022. www.sgo.org/resources/revisions-to-fda-approvals-for-parp-inhibitors/

65. Scambia G et al., Olaparib as treatment versus nonplatinum chemotherapy in patients with platinum-sensitive relapsed ovarian cancer: Phase III SOLO3 study final overall survival results. *J Clin Oncol*, 2024;**43**:1408–17.

History and Current Role of Immunotherapy in Ovarian Cancer Treatment

5

Stephanie Chow and Oliver Dorigo

5.1 INTRODUCTION

Ovarian cancer is the seventh most prevalent cancer among women globally and the leading cause of death from gynecologic malignancies. It is characterized by its insidious onset with vague symptoms, leading to diagnosis at advanced stages, when curative treatment is challenging. The current standard of care for ovarian cancer involves surgery followed by chemotherapy with platinum-based regimens. However, despite initially favorable responses to treatment, the majority of patients experience disease recurrence, eventually developing resistance to chemotherapy. These factors pose significant challenges to long-term disease control and survival.

DOI: 10.1201/9781003312475-5

The limitations of conventional therapies in managing advanced and recurrent ovarian cancer underscore the urgent need for innovative treatment modalities. Immunotherapy has revolutionized cancer treatment paradigms by exploiting the host's immune system to recognize and eliminate cancer cells. Unlike traditional therapies that directly target tumor cells, immunotherapy aims to enhance the body's own immune response, leading to durable antitumor effects and potentially fewer adverse effects compared to chemotherapy and radiation.

Ovarian cancer's immunogenic nature, characterized by tumor-infiltrating lymphocytes and immune evasion mechanisms, provides a strong rationale for exploring immunotherapy in this malignancy. Furthermore, the success of immunotherapeutic agents in other solid tumors, such as melanoma and lung cancer, has fueled interest in evaluating their efficacy and safety in gynecologic malignancies. Here, we will explore the historical evolution, current landscape, and future prospects of immunotherapy in the management of ovarian cancer.

5.2 HISTORICAL PERSPECTIVE OF IMMUNOTHERAPY

The concept of immunotherapy dates back to the late 19th century when an orthopedic surgeon, Dr. William Coley, observed tumor regression following acute bacterial infections in cancer patients. This observation led him to hypothesize that the immune system could be stimulated to attack cancer cells. Experimenting with this idea, he injected live and inactivated *Streptococcus pyogenes* and *Serratia marcescens*, later known as *"Coley's toxins,"* into sarcoma sites and observed tumor shrinkage, thus laying the groundwork for cancer immunology (1).

In the following decades, advancements in understanding immune mechanisms, such as T-cell activation and immune checkpoints, paved the way for more targeted immunotherapies. The advent of monoclonal antibodies (mAbs) (2) – molecules engineered to serve as substitute antibodies that can restore, enhance, or mimic the body's own immune system – in the 1970s marked a significant milestone in cancer treatment. In the 1970s, César Milstein and Georges Köhler pioneered the development of the hybridoma technology for the production of mAbs (3). This groundbreaking achievement earned them the Nobel Prize in Physiology or Medicine in 1984 and laid the foundation for the development of therapeutic antibodies for cancer treatment. In 1997, rituximab, a chimeric anti-CD20 antibody, became the first therapeutic mAb to receive regulatory approval for the treatment of non-Hodgkin's lymphoma, marking a major milestone in cancer immunotherapy.

Since then, medical and technological advances have led to the development of a diverse array of mAbs targeting various cancer-associated antigens, allowing immunotherapy to evolve from non-specific immunostimulants to sophisticated immune checkpoint inhibitors and adoptive cell therapies. The discovery of immune checkpoints, including cytotoxic T-lymphocyte-associated antigen 4 (CTLA-4) and programmed cell death protein 1 (PD-1), has revolutionized cancer treatment by lifting the brakes on immune responses against tumors. In 2011, ipilimumab, which targets CTLA-4 in metastatic melanoma, became the first immune checkpoint inhibitor to gain regulatory approval. This landmark approval ushered in a new era of cancer immunotherapy and sparked intense interest in targeting other immune checkpoints for cancer treatment. Subsequent clinical trials demonstrated the efficacy of PD-1/PD-L1 inhibitors in various solid tumors, leading to their widespread adoption in clinical practice. More recently, the development of chimeric antigen receptor (CAR) T-cell therapy has shown remarkable success in hematologic malignancies, paving the way for its application in solid tumors, including ovarian cancer (See further Figure 5.1).

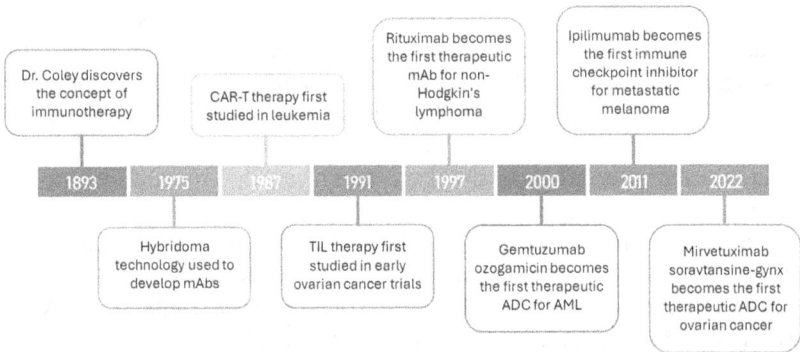

FIGURE 5.1   Timeline of major developments in immunotherapy: ADC, antibody drug conjugate; AML, acute myeloid leukemia; mAb, monoclonal antibody; TIL, tumor-infiltrating lymphocyte.

5.3 BIOMARKERS AND PATIENT SELECTION

Identifying predictive biomarkers is crucial for optimizing patient selection, guiding treatment decisions, and maximizing the efficacy of immunotherapy in ovarian cancer. Several biomarkers have been investigated to predict immunotherapeutic response in ovarian cancer, including programmed death-ligand 1 (PD-L1) expression, tumor-infiltrating lymphocytes (TILs), tumor mutational burden (TMB), and immune gene signatures (4).

PD-L1 expression on tumor cells and immune infiltrates has been extensively studied as a potential predictive biomarker for positive response to immune checkpoint inhibitors targeting the PD-1/PD-L1 axis. High PD-L1 expression has been associated with improved response rates and survival outcomes in various solid tumors, including ovarian cancer (5). However, PD-L1 expression alone may not be sufficient to predict response to immunotherapy, as some patients with low or absent PD-L1 expression still derive clinical benefits from treatment.

TILs, particularly cytotoxic CD8+ T cells, are critical in mediating antitumor immune responses and are indicative of an active immune microenvironment. High levels of TILs have been associated with better prognosis and improved responses to immunotherapy in ovarian cancer (6). Assessing TIL density and distribution within the tumor microenvironment may serve as a predictive biomarker for immunotherapy response and guide treatment selection in ovarian cancer patients.

TMB refers to the total number of somatic mutations within the tumor genome and is indicative of tumor immunogenicity. High TMB has been associated with increased neoantigen production and enhanced T cell recognition, leading to improved response to immune checkpoint inhibitors in multiple cancer types (7). In ovarian cancer, high TMB has been correlated with improved progression-free survival and overall survival in patients treated with immunotherapy, highlighting its potential utility as a predictive biomarker (8).

Advances in genomics and transcriptomics have enabled the identification of immune gene signatures that correlate with response to immunotherapy. These signatures provide insights into the immune landscape of tumors and help predict which patients are more likely to benefit from immunotherapy. However, the clinical utility of these signatures in ovarian cancer is still under investigation, and further research is needed to validate their predictive value in larger patient cohorts.

Predictive biomarkers hold immense promise for optimizing patient selection and improving outcomes with immunotherapy in ovarian cancer. Further research is warranted to validate these biomarkers in larger patient cohorts, establish standardized assays for biomarker assessment, and elucidate the complex interplay between the tumor microenvironment and immune responses.

5.4 IMMUNOTHERAPEUTIC STRATEGIES IN OVARIAN CANCER

5.4.1 Immune Checkpoint Inhibitors

Immune checkpoint inhibitors have become a cornerstone of cancer immunotherapy, with several agents approved for treating various malignancies, including melanoma, lung, breast, bladder, and renal cancers. These agents target inhibitory pathways that regulate T-cell activation and function, thereby enhancing antitumor immune responses. In ovarian cancer, immune checkpoint inhibitors have shown modest activity as monotherapy, prompting investigations into combination strategies to improve efficacy.

The PD-1/PD-L1 axis plays a crucial role in immune evasion by cancer cells by inhibiting T-cell activation and function, which reduces the immune system's ability to recognize and attack cancer cells. Blocking this pathway facilitates T-cell–mediated antitumor responses. Several clinical trials have investigated the efficacy and safety of this class of immunotherapeutic agents alone or in combination with standard therapies in ovarian cancer. For instance, the KEYNOTE-028, a phase Ib study, evaluated pembrolizumab, an anti-PD-1 antibody, in PD-L1–expressing advanced ovarian cancer (9). Pembrolizumab demonstrated durable responses in a subset of heavily pretreated patients, with an overall response rate (ORR) of 11.5% and 26.9% of patients achieving stable disease. Pembrolizumab was further investigated in the phase II KEYNOTE-100 study where patients with recurrent or advanced ovarian cancer previously treated with at least three lines of chemotherapy received pembrolizumab monotherapy until disease progression or toxicity (10), resulting in an ORR of 8% and a disease control rate (DCR) of 37%. Subgroup analyses suggested that patients with higher levels of PD-L1 expression may derive greater benefit from pembrolizumab treatment.

Combining chemotherapy with immunotherapy holds promise for synergistic antitumor effects, as chemotherapy-induced cell death can potentiate immune responses and enhance the efficacy of immunotherapeutic agents.

Initial studies, particularly in the frontline setting, have shown modest responses. The IMagyn050 trial investigated the combination of the anti-PD-L1 antibody atezolizumab with platinum-based chemotherapy followed by maintenance atezolizumab in patients with newly diagnosed advanced ovarian cancer (11). Although there was no significant difference in progression-free survival (PFS) in the intention-to-treat population, the trial demonstrated significantly improved PFS in the PD-L1 positive cohort (hazard ratio [HR] 0.80; 95% CI 0.65-0.99; P = 0.038). Another phase III study, the JAVELIN Ovarian 100 trial, investigated the anti-PD-L1 antibody, avelumab, in combination with and as maintenance therapy in previously untreated advanced epithelial ovarian cancer (12). Unfortunately, the study was stopped due to futility.

Avelumab was also investigated in recurrent platinum-resistant or refractory setting. In JAVELIN Ovarian 200, patients were randomized to either avelumab, avelumab plus pegylated liposomal doxorubicin (PLD), or PLD alone (13). Although the trial did not meet its primary endpoint of improved PFS in the avelumab arms compared to PLD alone, subgroup analyses suggested potential benefits in certain patient subsets, such as those with PD-L1-positive tumors. This trial underscored the challenges of patient selection and the importance of identifying predictive biomarkers to guide immunotherapy treatment decisions in ovarian cancer.

With the introduction of poly (adenosine diphosphate-ribose) polymerase (PARP) inhibitors, the armamentarium for ovarian cancer further evolved. PARP inhibitors work by blocking the enzyme PARP, which is involved in repairing DNA damage in cells. Inhibiting PARP prevents ovarian cancer cells, which often have defective DNA repair mechanisms, from repairing their DNA, triggering an antitumor immune response, leading to cell death and reduced tumor growth. In preclinical models, PARP inhibitors demonstrated synergistic interactions with immunotherapy (14). Combining targeted therapies with immunotherapy may overcome resistance mechanisms and enhance antitumor immune responses. The phase I–II trial, Topacio/KEYNOTE-162, evaluated the combination of the PARP inhibitor niraparib with pembrolizumab in platinum-resistant ovarian cancer (15). The ORR was 18% with a DCR of 65%, with ORRs consistent across multiple subgroups based on platinum sensitivity, prior bevacizumab treatment, and BRCA or homologous recombination deficiency (HRD) status. These encouraging response rates and durable clinical benefit demonstrate the potential synergy between PARP inhibition and immune checkpoint blockade in ovarian cancer, supporting further investigation in combination strategies targeting DNA repair defects and immune evasion mechanisms.

Cytotoxic T-lymphocyte-associated protein 4 (CTLA-4) is another immune checkpoint molecule that negatively regulates T cell activation. Blockade of CTLA-4 enhances T cell priming and effector function, leading to amplified antitumor immune responses (16). Preclinical studies have shown improved antitumor activity with dual checkpoint inhibition targeting CTLA-4 and PD-1 (17). In a phase II trial evaluated ipilimumab (anti-CTLA-4) and nivolumab (anti-PD-1) in recurrent/persistent ovarian cancer (18), patients were randomized to nivolumab or nivolumab plus ipilimumab treatment groups followed by maintenance nivolumab. The study demonstrated improved response rates with the combination therapy compared to nivolumab alone, 31.4% and 12.2%, respectively. In addition, there was extension of PFS (3.9 and 2 months, respectively; HR 0.528) with nivolumab plus ipilimumab. While immune checkpoint inhibitors have shown promise in the treatment of ovarian cancer, additional studies are warranted determine optimal combinations, efficacy, and improved outcomes.

5.4.2 Adoptive Cell Therapy

Adoptive cell therapy involves the *ex vivo* expansion and infusion of autologous or allogeneic immune cells engineered to recognize and target tumor antigens. The first clinical application of adoptive cell therapy was described in 1988 for the treatment of metastatic melanoma (19). The two major approaches are TIL therapy and CAR-T cell therapy.

5.4.3 Tumor-Infiltrating Lymphocytes (TILs)

TIL therapy involves the isolation, expansion, and reinfusion of tumor-reactive lymphocytes derived from surgically resected tumors. These lymphocytes are thought to possess ongoing anti-tumor responses and TIL therapy has shown promise in some types of cancer, such as melanoma. Preclinical and early-phase clinical studies have shown promising results with TIL therapy in ovarian cancer, warranting further investigation in larger cohorts. Beginning in the early 1990s, the earliest clinical studies of TILs in ovarian cancer demonstrated complete and partial responses in metastatic disease (20) with significantly increased disease-free survival rates (21). More recent studies have investigated combinations with other therapeutics. Kverneland et al. treated six late-stage metastatic ovarian cancer patients with TILs combined with ipilimumab and nivolumab (22). One patient achieved a partial response and five had up to 12 months of disease stabilization. The exact mechanism of action of TILs in immunotherapy for ovarian cancer is not fully understood, but it is thought to involve the recognition and elimination of tumor cells by the re-infused TILs, mediated by their ability to recognize tumor-specific antigens presented on the surface of cancer cells. Additionally, TIL therapy may also help to overcome the immunosuppressive environment within the tumor, allowing for a more effective immune response against the cancer. Larger-scale studies are needed to further elucidate the efficacy, safety, and long-term outcomes of TIL therapy in ovarian cancer as well as identify key biomarkers that predict favorable responses.

5.4.4 CAR-T Cell Therapy

CAR-T therapy is a type of immunotherapy that involves engineering a patient's own T cells to express synthetic receptors, termed chimeric antigen receptors (CARs), that recognize tumor-associated antigens. CAR-T therapy was introduced in the experimental setting in 1987, with ongoing research leading to regulatory approval of tisagenlecleucel as third-line treatment for B-cell acute lymphoblastic leukemia. While CAR-T therapy has shown remarkable success in treating hematological malignancies, its application in solid tumors, including ovarian cancer, is more challenging. Solid tumors present a more complex microenvironment, characterized by physical barriers, immunosuppressive factors, and heterogeneous antigen expression which makes it more difficult for CAR-T cells to effectively infiltrate the tumor and sustain their anti-tumor activity. Despite these hurdles, research is ongoing to optimize CAR-T therapy for ovarian cancer, and multiple CAR-T products are under investigation for the treatment of ovarian cancer in varying stages of development. The most common CAR-T targets include AMHR2, ANXA2, BCMA, B7-H3, CD19, CD20, CD22, CD30, CD38, CD123, CGRP, Claudin, EGFR, EpCAM, FOLR1, GD2 TROP-2, HER2, mesothelin, MUC1, MUC16, PD-L1, SLAMF7, and VEGF-R (23, 24). Preclinical and clinical efforts are ongoing to discover optimal CAR-T target antigens that result in improved antitumor efficacy while minimizing toxicity.

5.4.5 Cancer Vaccines

Cancer vaccines are a type of immunotherapy that stimulates the body's own immune system to recognize and mount an immune response against tumor-specific antigens. Unlike traditional vaccines that prevent diseases, cancer vaccines are designed to treat existing cancer or prevent its recurrence. In 1891, when Dr. William Coley injected live and inactivated *Streptococcus pyogenes* and *Serratia marcescens* (25) intratumorally, he was in effect evaluating the first concept of cancer vaccines. In the last three decades, there have been massive improvements in vaccine development, with various vaccine platforms currently being evaluated including dendritic cell vaccines, peptide-based vaccines, and biovectors (26).

Dendritic cells (DC) are specialized immune cells that play a crucial role in presenting antigens to T cells, activating them to recognize and eliminate cancer cells. In DC vaccinations, DCs are isolated from patients, manipulated *ex vivo* to generate and activate DCs loaded with tumor antigens, and then re-infused into patients to stimulate immune responses. DCs are typically loaded with either recombinant peptides or tumor lysate to harness antigen-specific cytotoxic T cell responses. DC vaccines in ovarian cancer have demonstrated encouraging clinical benefits and safety profiles in early phase trials (27). More recently, Tanyi et al. investigated personalized vaccines generated by pulsing autologous dendritic cells with oxidized autologous whole-tumor cell lysate (28). The vaccine was injected into the lymph nodes of ovarian cancer patients, inducing T cell responses to the tumor antigens and to previously unrecognized mutated neoantigens. These observations inspired additional investigations into the combination of vaccine-primed T cells and adoptive cell therapy. In a phase I, follow-on study, 19 patients were administered further treatment with adoptive cell transfer of vaccine-primed autologous peripheral blood T cells and bevacizumab (29). The median OS was 14.2 months, with restoration of preexisting immunity to neopeptides and establishment of responses to new neopeptides.

Peptide vaccines consist of short amino acid sequences derived from tumor-associated antigens, administered to stimulate T-cell responses. These peptides are selected based on their ability to bind to major histocompatibility complex molecules and activate T cells. Several peptide vaccines targeting ovarian cancer-associated antigens, such as HER2/neu, NY-ESO-1, and WT1, have been investigated in preclinical and early clinical studies. While peptide vaccines offer advantages such as ease of production and administration, their efficacy in inducing robust and durable antitumor immune responses remains a subject of ongoing research. Recent evidence suggests the combination of peptide vaccines and immune checkpoint inhibitors results in improved antitumor immune responses. Eleven patients were treated in a phase I study of the Wilms' Tumor 1 (WT1) peptide vaccine (galinpepimut-S) in combination with nivolumab for recurrent ovarian cancer (30). The study reported a 91% T cell response to WT1 peptides, and the 1-year PFS rate was 70% in patients who received more than two treatments of the vaccine/immunotherapy combination.

Oncolytic viruses are genetically engineered to selectively infect and destroy cancer cells while sparing normal tissues. They are designed to replicate within cancer cells, causing them to lyse and release tumor antigens, which can then stimulate an immune response against the disease. In addition to the direct lysis of cancer cells, oncolytic viruses also exert their antitumor effects through the induction of immunogenic cell death and activation of innate and adaptive immune responses. The viruses can also serve as a therapeutic vector to deliver exogenous genes to amplify immune responses and restore antitumor immunity. Key oncolytic viruses under investigation for ovarian cancer include modified vaccinia virus, adenovirus, and herpes simplex virus. Clinical trials are underway, exploring both single oncolytic virus therapy and combination therapies with other treatments (31). Early studies utilizing Olvi-Vec, an oncolytic vaccinia virus-based immunotherapy, demonstrated an ORR of 54% and median PFS of 11.0 months in heavily pretreated platinum-resistant/refractory ovarian cancer (32). Given these promising results, the combination of Olvi-Vec and chemotherapy is being investigated in the phase III OnPrime/GOG-3076 study to determine the efficacy of virus-mediated immune activation and re-sensitization of tumor cells to chemotherapy (33).

Despite progress in multiple clinical trials, challenges remain in optimizing the clinical efficacy of cancer vaccines for ovarian cancer. The heterogeneity of ovarian cancer makes it difficult to identify universal tumor antigens that can be targeted by vaccines and cancer cells may evolve to lose the expression of targeted antigens, allowing them to evade immune recognition and rendering vaccines ineffective (antigen escape). Additionally, the immunosuppressive tumor microenvironment in ovarian cancer patients can dampen the effectiveness of these vaccines. Ongoing research is therefore directed at improving vaccine formulations, identifying synergistic combinations with other therapies, and overcoming immunosuppression to enhance the antitumor immune response.

5.4.6 Antibody-drug Conjugates

Antibody-drug conjugates (ADCs) represent a promising class of targeted cancer therapies designed to deliver cytotoxic drugs directly to tumor cells while sparing normal tissues, thereby reducing systemic toxicity. The concept of ADCs originated from the pioneering work of scientists in the late 20th century who sought to combine the specificity of monoclonal antibodies (mAbs) with the cytotoxic potency of chemotherapy drugs. They generally consist of three main components: an antibody that specifically recognizes a tumor-associated antigen, a cytotoxic drug, and a linker that connects the antibody to the drug. The development of hybridoma technology by César Milstein and Georges Köhler in the 1970s facilitated the production of monoclonal antibodies, laying the groundwork for the creation of ADCs.

In 2000, the first ADC to receive regulatory approval was gemtuzumab ozogamicin, targeting CD33 for acute myeloid leukemia. This milestone demonstrated the clinical potential of ADCs in delivering potent cytotoxic payloads selectively to cancer cells. Subsequent advancements in linker chemistry and payload selection led to the development of next-generation ADCs with improved stability, efficacy, and safety profiles.

In ovarian cancer, ongoing research efforts are focused on the development of novel ADCs targeting tumor-specific antigens, such as folate receptor alpha (FRα), mesothelin, and mucin-16 (CA-125). In 2022, accelerated regulatory approval was granted to mirvetuximab soravtansine-gynx (MIRV), an ADC–targeting FRα-positive, platinum-resistant ovarian cancer. The MIRASOL trial enrolled 453 ovarian cancer patients who had previously received one to three prior lines of chemotherapy, and were randomized to receive either MIRV or chemotherapy (34). Objective responses were higher in the MIRV group compared to the chemotherapy group (42.3% vs. 15.9%, respectively), and there was a statistically significant improvement in median OS (16.5 vs. 12.7 months; HR 0.67; 95% CI 0.50-0.89).

Currently, there are more than 15 ADCs under preclinical investigation for ovarian cancer, with some being evaluated in early-phase clinical trials showing promising results (35). These investigations are crucial for understanding the full potential of ADCs in ovarian cancer treatment and for identifying new targets and strategies to enhance their effectiveness.

5.5 FUTURE DIRECTIONS AND EMERGING THERAPIES

5.5.1 Novel Immunotherapeutic Approaches

Advances in cancer immunology and molecular biology continue to drive the development of novel immunotherapeutic approaches for ovarian cancer. Targeting additional immune checkpoints, modulating the tumor microenvironment, and exploiting synthetic biology tools are among the strategies being explored to enhance the efficacy of immunotherapy in this malignancy.

5.5.2 Bispecific Antibodies

Bispecific antibodies are engineered molecules that simultaneously bind to two different antigens, typically a tumor-associated antigen and an immune cell receptor, to enhance tumor recognition and immune mediated cytotoxicity. The concept of bispecific antibodies emerged from the desire to enhance the specificity and potency of antibody-based therapies by redirecting immune effector cells, such as T cells or natural killer cells, to tumor cells. The development of bispecific antibodies began in the 1980s with the advent of hybrid hybridoma technology, which enabled the generation of bispecific antibodies with defined specificities. Early bispecific antibodies, such as blinatumomab targeting CD19 and CD3 in acute lymphoblastic leukemia, demonstrated proof-of-concept for redirecting T cells to tumor cells and inducing tumor regression.

In ovarian cancer, bispecific antibodies targeting MUC16 and CD3 are being investigated in early-phase clinical trials (NCT03564340). These bispecific antibodies aim to facilitate contact between T cells and cancer cells, unleashing the cytotoxic potential of immune effector cells and overcoming immunosuppressive mechanisms within the tumor microenvironment, offering a potentially more effective and targeted approach compared to traditional monoclonal antibody therapies. Additional preclinical studies are underway, investigating CD73xEpCAM, PD-1xVEGF, CLDN6xCD3, and others (36–38). These studies provide a rationale for the clinical development of next-generation immunotherapies with enhanced specificity and potency, offering new therapeutic options for ovarian cancer patients refractory to conventional treatments.

5.5.3 Combination Strategies Beyond Traditional Immunotherapy

Combining immunotherapy with other treatment modalities, such as targeted therapies and radiation therapies, represents a promising approach to overcome resistance mechanisms and improve treatment outcomes in ovarian cancer. Rational selection of combination partners and optimization of treatment regimens are critical for maximizing therapeutic synergy and minimizing toxicity.

5.5.4 PARP Inhibitors and Immune Checkpoint Inhibitors

To reduce recurrence risk in ovarian cancer, maintenance therapy with a PARP inhibitor and/or bevacizumab has become a standard of care option in therapy. The combination treatment using immune checkpoint inhibitors and PARP inhibitors have been shown to provide synergistic effects (39). DUO-O was a phase III trial investigating the efficacy and safety of triplet maintenance treatment with bevacizumab plus olaparib and the immunotherapy durvalumab. The study found a greater PFS with triplet maintenance treatment compared to bevacizumab monotherapy in patients with newly diagnosed advanced stage ovarian cancer without tumor BRCA mutations (40). The combination therapy also showed a favorable safety profile, with manageable adverse events. Though the initial results were encouraging, final analysis is pending and additional studies are needed to explore combination strategies that achieve more durable responses in a broader patient population.

5.5.5 Immunotherapy and Radiation

Ionizing radiation therapy has long been known to induce DNA damage, resulting in cancer cell death. However, the concept of radiation modulating the tumor microenvironment to enhance immune responses has been increasingly recognized. The synergy of immunotherapy with radiation treatment is multifaceted. Radiation can induce immunogenic cell death, releasing tumor antigens that can prime the immune system, and can enhance the infiltration of immune cells into the tumor microenvironment. Preclinical studies have shown that the immunogenic cell death from radiation exposes tumor-associated antigens, which promote T-cell responses, making it an attractive partner for combination with immunotherapy (41). Despite early evidence of the synergistic effects of radiation therapy and immunotherapy in ovarian cancer, more studies are needed to evaluate this combination in humans. Clinical trials attempting to investigate this have unfortunately terminated (NCT03277482) or closed due to poor accrual (NCT03312114).

5.5.6 Pioneering Studies in Ovarian Cancer Immunotherapy

Innovative research is currently being conducted using the CRISPR-Cas9 gene-editing system, which holds the promise of enabling more precise alterations of gene function for therapeutic applications, thereby allowing the development of more effective and safer CAR-T cell therapies. This versatile gene-editing method is being applied to construct CAR-T cells and T cell receptor T (TCR-T) cells, inhibit immune checkpoint signaling pathways, and identify new targets for ovarian cancer immunotherapy (42). Additionally, the versatility of CRISPR-Cas9 allows for the development of personalized CAR-T cell therapies tailored to individual patients' tumor profiles, further enhancing their therapeutic potential. As this field continues to grow, it is poised to revolutionize the current landscape of cancer therapy and bring forth more precise gene function modification for therapeutic use.

5.6 CONCLUSION

Immunotherapy has emerged as a promising therapeutic approach in ovarian cancer, offering the potential for durable responses, reduced adverse effects, and improved survival outcomes in select subsets of patients. Key immunotherapeutic strategies, including immune checkpoint inhibitors, adoptive cell therapy, cancer vaccines, and oncolytic viruses, have shown encouraging results in clinical trials. Ongoing efforts are focused on optimizing treatment regimens, identifying predictive biomarkers, and overcoming resistance mechanisms. The integration of immunotherapy into the treatment landscape of ovarian cancer requires multidisciplinary collaboration and personalized treatment approaches tailored to individual patient characteristics and tumor biology. Biomarker-driven patient selection and rational combination strategies hold promise for maximizing the efficacy of immunotherapy and improving patient outcomes in this challenging disease. Despite the progress made in the field of immunotherapy for ovarian cancer, several challenges and unanswered questions remain, including the identification of reliable predictive biomarkers, optimization of combination therapies, and management of treatment-related toxicities without compromising treatment efficacy. Continued research is essential to address these challenges and unlock the full potential of immunotherapy in transforming the standard of care for ovarian cancer patients.

REFERENCES

1. Coley WB. The treatment of malignant tumors by repeated inoculations of erysipelas. With a report of ten original cases. 1893. *Clin Orthop Relat Res* 1991;(262):3–11.
2. Weiner LM et al. Monoclonal antibodies: versatile platforms for cancer immunotherapy. *Nat Rev Immunol* 2010;**10**(5):317–27.
3. Kohler G, Milstein C. Continuous cultures of fused cells secreting antibody of predefined specificity. *Nature* 1975;**256**(5517):495–7.
4. Konecny GE *et al.* Prognostic and therapeutic relevance of molecular subtypes in high-grade serous ovarian cancer. *J Natl Cancer Inst* 2014;**106**(10).
5. Hamanishi J *et al.* Safety and antitumor activity of Anti-PD-1 antibody, nivolumab, in patients with platinum-resistant ovarian cancer. *J Clin Oncol* 2015;**33**(34):4015–22.
6. Zhang L *et al.* Intratumoral T cells, recurrence, and survival in epithelial ovarian cancer. *N Engl J Med* 2003;**348**(3):203–13.

7. Yarchoan M et al. Tumor mutational burden and response rate to PD-1 inhibition. *N Engl J Med* 2017;**377**(25):2500–1.

8. Mi JL et al. Interactions between tumor mutation burden and immune infiltration in ovarian cancer. *Int J Clin Exp Pathol* 2020;**13**(10):2513–23.

9. Varga A *et al.* Pembrolizumab in patients with programmed death ligand 1-positive advanced ovarian cancer: Analysis of KEYNOTE-028. *Gynecol Oncol* 2019;**152**(2):243–50.

10. Matulonis UA *et al.* Antitumor activity and safety of pembrolizumab in patients with advanced recurrent ovarian cancer: results from the phase II KEYNOTE-100 study. *Ann Oncol* 2019;**30**(7):1080–7.

11. Moore KN *et al.* Atezolizumab, bevacizumab, and chemotherapy for newly diagnosed stage III or IV ovarian cancer: Placebo-controlled randomized phase III trial (IMagyn050/GOG 3015/ENGOT-OV39). *J Clin Oncol* 2021;**39**(17):1842–55.

12. Monk BJ *et al.* Chemotherapy with or without avelumab followed by avelumab maintenance versus chemotherapy alone in patients with previously untreated epithelial ovarian cancer (JAVELIN Ovarian 100): an open-label, randomised, phase 3 trial. *Lancet Oncol* 2021;**22**(9):1275–89.

13. Pujade-Lauraine E *et al.* Avelumab alone or in combination with chemotherapy versus chemotherapy alone in platinum-resistant or platinum-refractory ovarian cancer (JAVELIN Ovarian 200): an open-label, three-arm, randomised, phase 3 study. *Lancet Oncol* 2021;**22**(7):1034–46.

14. Shen J *et al.* PARPi triggers the STING-dependent immune response and enhances the therapeutic efficacy of immune checkpoint blockade independent of BRCAness. *Cancer Res* 2019;**79**(2):311–9.

15. Konstantinopoulos PA *et al.* Single-arm phases 1 and 2 trial of niraparib in combination with pembrolizumab in patients with recurrent platinum-resistant ovarian carcinoma. *JAMA Oncol* 2019;**5**(8):1141–9.

16. Seidel JA et al. Anti-PD-1 and anti-CTLA-4 therapies in cancer: Mechanisms of action, efficacy, and limitations. *Front Oncol* 2018;**8**:86.

17. Curran MA et al. PD-1 and CTLA-4 combination blockade expands infiltrating T cells and reduces regulatory T and myeloid cells within B16 melanoma tumors. *Proc Natl Acad Sci USA* 2010;**107**(9):4275–80.

18. Zamarin D *et al.* Randomized phase II trial of nivolumab versus nivolumab and ipilimumab for recurrent or persistent ovarian cancer: An NRG oncology study. *J Clin Oncol* 2020;**38**(16):1814–23.

19. Rosenberg SA *et al.* Use of tumor-infiltrating lymphocytes and interleukin-2 in the immunotherapy of patients with metastatic melanoma. A preliminary report. *N Engl J Med* 1988;**319**(25):1676–80.

20. Aoki Y *et al.* Use of adoptive transfer of tumor-infiltrating lymphocytes alone or in combination with cisplatin-containing chemotherapy in patients with epithelial ovarian cancer. *Cancer Res* 1991;**51**(7):1934–9.

21. Fujita K *et al.* Prolonged disease-free period in patients with advanced epithelial ovarian cancer after adoptive transfer of tumor-infiltrating lymphocytes. *Clin Cancer Res* 1995;**1**(5):501–7.

22. Kverneland AH *et al.* Adoptive cell therapy in combination with checkpoint inhibitors in ovarian cancer. *Oncotarget* 2020;**11**(22):2092–105.

23. Nasiri F et al. CAR-T cell immunotherapy for ovarian cancer: Hushing the silent killer. *Front Immunol* 2023;**14**:1302307.
24. Zhang XW et al. CAR-T cells in the treatment of ovarian cancer: A promising cell therapy. *Biomolecules* 2023;**13**(3).
25. McCarthy EF. The toxins of William B. Coley and the treatment of bone and soft-tissue sarcomas. *Iowa Orthop J* 2006;**26**:154–8.
26. Chow S et al. Development of Therapeutic Vaccines for Ovarian Cancer. *Vaccines (Basel)* 2020;**8**(4).
27. Guo Q et al. Advanced clinical trials of dendritic cell vaccines in ovarian cancer. *J Investig Med* 2020;**68**(7):1223–7.
28. Tanyi JL *et al.* Personalized cancer vaccine effectively mobilizes antitumor T cell immunity in ovarian cancer. *Sci Transl Med* 2018;**10**(436).
29. Bobisse S *et al.* A phase 1 trial of adoptive transfer of vaccine-primed autologous circulating T cells in ovarian cancer. *Nat Cancer* 2023;**4**(10):1410–7.
30. Manning-Geist BL *et al.* Phase I study of a multivalent WT1 peptide vaccine (Galinpepimut-S) in combination with nivolumab in patients with WT1-expressing ovarian cancer in second or third remission. *Cancers (Basel)* 2023; **15**(5).
31. Pampeno C et al. sindbis virus vaccine platform: A promising oncolytic virus-mediated approach for ovarian cancer treatment. *Int J Mol Sci* 2024;**25**(5).
32. Holloway RW *et al.* Clinical activity of olvimulogene nanivacirepvec-primed immunochemotherapy in heavily pretreated patients with platinum-resistant or platinum-refractory ovarian cancer: the nonrandomized phase 2 VIRO-15 clinical trial. *JAMA Oncol* 2023;**9**(7):903–8.
33. Holloway RW *et al.* A phase III, multicenter, randomized study of olvimulogene nanivacirepvec followed by platinum-doublet chemotherapy and bevacizumab compared with platinum-doublet chemotherapy and bevacizumab in women with platinum-resistant/refractory ovarian cancer. *Int J Gynecol Cancer* 2023;**33**(9):1458–63.
34. Moore KN *et al.* Mirvetuximab Soravtansine in FRalpha-positive, platinum-resistant ovarian cancer. *N Engl J Med* 2023;**389**(23):2162–74.
35. Manzano A, Ocana A. Antibody-drug conjugates: A promising novel therapy for the treatment of ovarian cancer. *Cancers (Basel)* 2020;**12**(8).
36. Ploeg EM *et al.* A novel bispecific antibody for EpCAM-directed inhibition of the CD73/adenosine immune checkpoint in ovarian cancer. *Cancers (Basel)* 2023;**15**(14).
37. Lingying W et al. A phase 1b/II clinical study of AK112, a PD-1/VEGF bispecific antibody, in combination with olaparib in BRCA germline wild-type platinum sensitive recurrent ovarian cancer. *J ImmunoTherapy Cancer* 2021;**9**.
38. Rucker J et al. Development of CTIM-76, a highly specific Claudin 6 bispecific antibody for treatment of ovarian cancer [abstract]. *Cancer Res*;**83**: (7_Suppl):Abstract 1865.
39. Musacchio L *et al.* Combining PARP inhibition and immune checkpoint blockade in ovarian cancer patients: a new perspective on the horizon? *ESMO Open* 2022;**7**(4):100536.

40. Harter P et al. Durvalumab with paclitaxel/carboplatin and bevacizumab followed by maintenance durvalumab, bevacizumab and olaparib in patients with newly diagnosed advanced ovarian cancer without a tumor BRCA1/BRCA2 mutation: Results from the randomized, placebo-controlled phase III DUO-O/ENGOT-ov46/AGO-OVAR 23/GOG-3025 trial. 2023 ASCO Annual Meeting. Abstract LBA5506.
41. Herrera FG et al. Rational combinations of immunotherapy with radiotherapy in ovarian cancer. *Lancet Oncol* 2019;**20**(8):e417–e33.
42. He ZY *et al.* In Vivo Ovarian Cancer Gene Therapy Using CRISPR-Cas9. *Hum Gene Ther* 2018;**29**(2):223–33.

The History and Current Role of Perioperative Care and Prehabilitation in Ovarian Cancer

6

Marlene Misu Lee and Jalid Sehouli

6.1 INTRODUCTION

Cytoreductive surgery is often a key component of first-line treatment for ovarian cancer, typically combined with platinum-based chemotherapy and, in many cases, followed by maintenance therapy (1).

Most ovarian cancer cases are diagnosed at an advanced stage with a high tumor burden (1). Optimal surgical treatment is essential since a critical determinant for survival is complete macroscopic tumor resection. To achieve this, multi-visceral resection and operating across multiple compartments, including the pelvis is often necessary (2). The increased technical complexity of surgery across multiple compartments, as well as operating in the pelvis, is associated with increased morbidity (1, 3).

DOI: 10.1201/9781003312475-6

In addition to surgical expertise, the quality of perioperative care plays an important role in the treatment success (4). Perioperative management seeks to alleviate the stress response caused by surgery, support physical function, and optimize recovery by implementing several small interventions combined into a comprehensive care pathway over the pre-, intra-, and postoperative period (5, 6). Perioperative management presents a more holistic approach to patient care, aiming to improve care beyond the operating room throughout the entire patient journey from first diagnosis to full postoperative recovery (4).

In the past, perioperative care was reactive, addressing symptoms or complications as they appeared. Patients spent prolonged times fasting and resting, further contributing to metabolic disturbances and stress responses caused by surgery (7). With the advancements in surgical and anesthesiologic management enabling more elaborate surgical procedures in an aging population with increasingly complex medical histories, there has been a growing recognition of the need for coordinated and structured care to support recovery (4, 5).

Initially known as fast-track rehabilitation, which focused on accelerating discharge from the hospital, perioperative care pathways have evolved into Enhanced Recovery After Surgery (ERAS), shifting the focus to a more comprehensive view on optimizing recovery (8). ERAS protocols were first developed for colorectal surgery and have since been adapted across various specialties, including gynecology and gynecologic oncology, showing measurable benefits such as reduced length of hospital stay and reduced complication rates (2, 3).

More recently, prehabilitation has emerged as an extension of perioperative care (9). It aims to proactively enhance patients' resilience ahead of surgery, in order to better withstand surgical stress and improve recovery (4). This concept is especially relevant for older or frail patients who are more susceptible to surgical stress and face an increased risk of complications (10, 11).

This chapter explores the historical development of perioperative care in gynecologic oncology, with a particular focus on ERAS and prehabilitation. It provides a perspective on how these advancements have shaped the current standard practice and explores potential future directions.

6.2 THE SIGNIFICANCE OF PERIOPERATIVE MANAGEMENT IN OVARIAN CANCER CARE

Cytoreductive surgery is a crucial component of the treatment of ovarian cancer. The complexity of these procedures can vary significantly, ranging from simpler operations such as completion hysterectomy and bilateral salpingo-oophorectomy to more extensive interventions involving peritoneal stripping, bowel resection, and upper abdominal surgery (1, 3). However, this type of complex surgery carries a significant risk of postoperative complications, which may delay subsequent therapeutic interventions, potentially contributing to worse overall outcomes (3).

Over the past decades, there have been significant improvements in surgical precision and anesthesiologic management, which led to a considerable decrease in surgery-related postoperative complications and better overall survival (5). However, general complications remain high, ranging between 20–60% (5). General complications refer to complications that are not primarily caused by surgical techniques but are significantly influenced by perioperative factors and include thromboembolic events and nosocomial infections, as well as organ dysfunction such as cardiologic or renal events (4, 5). In response to patient needs and surgical technology, there has been increasing emphasis on improving perioperative management (4, 5, 12).

Surgery triggers a significant stress response in the body, leading to hypermetabolism and catabolism by activating the immune system through inflammatory markers. These stress reactions can contribute to malnutrition and sarcopenia, which refers to the loss of muscle mass and optimal muscle function. They further contribute to weakened immune function, impaired wound healing, and organ dysfunction (1, 13).

The ERAS concept is based on the hypothesis that minimizing and better managing the physiological stress of surgery can optimize postoperative recovery (4, 5). ERAS protocols were designed to incorporate evidence-based interventions that help maintain homeostasis during the perioperative period and improve postoperative convalescence by minimizing disturbances in physiological function (4, 8).

Surgical stress causes metabolic disturbances, such as insulin resistance. However, within the ERAS pathway, several interventions contribute to ensuring metabolic stabilization (13). For instance, prolonged fasting periods before surgery should be avoided to reduce insulin resistance. Additionally, oral nutrition should be permitted up until 6 hours before surgery, and should be supported by ingesting a carbohydrate-rich drink before surgery (4, 7, 12). During the operation, blood glucose should be monitored and adjusted to avoid fluctuations (7). Continuing in the postoperative phase, early oral nutrition uptake contributes to insulin sensitivity and the resumption of gastrointestinal function (4, 7, 12). Fluid balance is also better maintained by avoiding aggressive bowel preparation before surgery and allowing patients to drink clear fluids up to two hours before surgery, preventing dehydration and electrolyte imbalances, as well as reducing the risk of renal stress (7, 14). Similarly, thoracic epidural analgesia in open surgery reduces the stress response through other mechanisms but with the same goal of metabolic stabilization (15). Furthermore, minimally invasive surgical techniques, if possible, decrease tissue trauma and

PRE - OP	INTRA - OP	POST - OP
• Patient education and counseling • Anemia correction • Smoking and alcohol cessation • Nutritional screening and optimization • Avoidance of prolonged fasting • Carbohydrate loading • Ommission of mechanical bowel preparation; if administered: mechanical bowel prep plus oral antibiotics • Avoidance of sedating pre-medication	• Use of minimally invasive surgical techniques, when appropriate • Standardized anesthetic protocol • Maintenance of normovolemia through goal-directed fluid management • Maintenance of normothermia • Antimicrobial prophylaxis (Chlorhexidine) • Antithrombotic prophylaxis (combined mechanical and medication) • Strict indication of drains and tubes	• Fluid management • Early mobilization • Early oral food intake • Multimodal, opioid-sparing analgesia • Early removal of drains and catheters • Prevention of nausea and vomiting

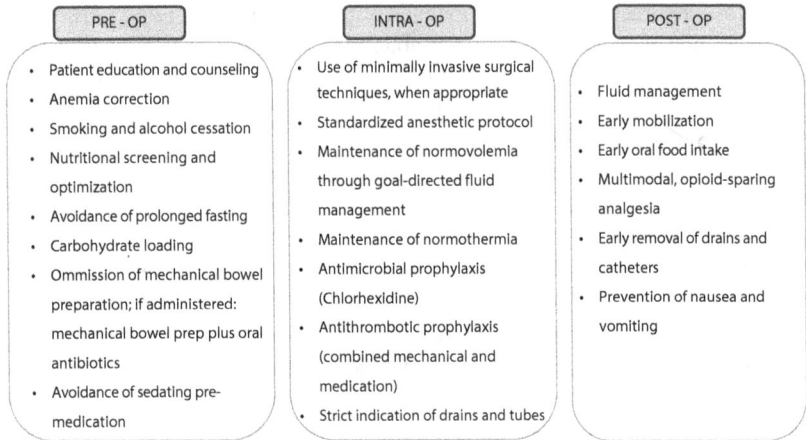

FIGURE 6.1   Key ERAS – items according to the ERAS®– Guidelines in Gynecologic Oncology (7, 9).

contribute to the limitation of inflammatory activation, which further decreases surgical stress (4, 7).

These multiple, targeted interventions all contribute to mitigating surgical stress and achieving a faster return to physiological function after surgery. The benefits of perioperative care pathways result from the consolidation of these multiple individual items that, when combined into a pathway, produce a synergistic effect, forming a comprehensive, multimodal approach to patient care (4, 5, 12).

The ERAS pathway represents a structured, evidence-based perioperative protocol. It was initially introduced in colorectal surgery and has since been widely adopted in various specialties, including gynecology and gynecologic oncology. In gynecologic oncology, where patients frequently present with heavy disease burden and undergo complex surgery, perioperative management is crucial for improving patient care (7, 9, 16) (Figure 6.1).

6.3 FROM THE EARLY STEPS OF FAST TRACK RECOVERY TO THE EMERGENCE OF ERAS

The concept of Enhanced Recovery after Surgery was first introduced in 1997 by Danish surgeon Henrik Kehlet under the name "fast-track surgery" (17).

While significant improvements had been made regarding surgery-related complications, primarily due to advances in surgical techniques and anesthesiologic management, general postoperative complications remained a persistent issue that needed to be further explored (17).

Kehlet argued that this was due to several factors. First, he emphasized the limitations of a unimodal view of complications. This entailed focusing on a single risk factor at a time. Examples include thromboembolic prophylaxis to prevent thrombosis and embolism or antimicrobial prophylaxis to reduce surgical site infections. Second, he pointed to the limitations of the traditional, compartmentalized orientation of medical specialties: surgeons focusing solely on surgical complications, such as surgical site infections and anastomotic leakage, and anesthesiologists focusing exclusively on the intraoperative and immediate postoperative management of cardiopulmonary function and fluid management, often neglecting the later phases of recovery. These two factors illustrate a fragmented, isolated view of complications and their management. Kehlet pointed out that postoperative complications are typically multicausal, which means that, most often, complications cannot be linked to one single issue but, more likely, several interrelating factors and causes that ultimately lead to a complication. This comprehensive view of complications requires a multimodal, interdisciplinary response involving collaboration across specialties (17).

Excluding complications that are directly linked to surgical or anesthetic techniques, most complications arise from the surgical stress response and the subsequent increased demand on various organ systems (13, 18). This perspective requires healthcare staff to adopt a broader, more integrated understanding of postoperative complications, spanning the entire postoperative period up until full recovery (17).

Kehlet argued that no unimodal approach or single intervention could sufficiently address these multicausal postoperative complications. Instead, he identified risk factors across the pre-, intra-, and postoperative phases that needed to be addressed collectively within a structured, multimodal care pathway (17).

In response, Kehlet proposed a new concept of a "multimodal recovery intervention," which included the reorganization of surgical wards into smaller "recovery units" focusing on early rehabilitation (17). The main components of these protocols were multimodal analgesia, early resumption of oral food intake, and early mobilization. These measures aimed to collectively mitigate the inflammatory and catabolic responses triggered by surgery. At the same time, recovery-impairing factors such as drains, tubes, urinary catheters, and prolonged fasting were limited (17). The idea was that drains, tubes, and urinary catheters that remain for extended periods increase the risk of infections while simultaneously limiting patients' mobilization (7).

Kehlet also proposed a multidisciplinary team approach involving surgeons, anesthesiologists, other health professionals such as physiotherapists, and, at the core, the patient (17). This approach was intended to put the patient at the center of care and engage and enable them to participate actively in their recovery journey. Moreover, the multidisciplinary approach supports a holistic view of complications and their management.

Furthermore, Kehlet suggested a centralization approach in which specialized centers should be formed where major abdominal surgeries would be performed (17).

Centralization was intended to support the development of high-level surgical expertise and provide infrastructure to assist the accelerated recovery approach further. These so-called "accelerated stay programs" were designed to reduce the length of hospital stays and healthcare costs (17, 19).

Many of the elements Kehlet suggested in this "multimodal recovery intervention" remain central to modern-day ERAS protocols. He advocated for transforming standard care by integrating individual interventions into a comprehensive care bundle, fostering collaboration among various medical specialties and healthcare professionals, actively involving patients in their treatment and recovery journey, implementing organizational changes, and establishing centralized care facilities (8, 17).

Following this publication, Kehlet published a trial showing a reduction in hospital stay by 3–8 days, with a mean hospital stay of 2 days, after elective open sigmoid resection in elderly patients (20). Even though the trial only included 16 patients, these results were considered groundbreaking at the time (8, 20).

A few years later, in 2001, Fast Track evolved to Enhanced Recovery After Surgery with the formation of the ERAS Study Group, co-founded by Ken Fearon (UK), Olle Ljunqvist (Sweden), Henrik Kehlet (Denmark), Arthur Revhaug (Norway), Maarten von Meyenfeldt (Netherlands) and Cornelius de Jong (Netherlands) (8). While Fast Track emphasized early discharge, the term *Enhanced Recovery* represented a shift in focus toward the patient's overall recovery process rather than only minimizing hospital stay (8).

The ERAS® Study Group soon discovered significant variation in practice between hospitals and a considerable gap between current routines and best practices supported by the literature. This led the group to a deeper investigation into how to transition from traditional care to evidence-based best practices (8, 21).

In 2005, the ERAS Study Group published the first recommendations for perioperative care in colonic resections. These are now considered the first formal consensus guidelines on perioperative care and the forerunner of the ERAS guidelines (21, 22). The ERAS Study Group also conducted several projects, implementing ERAS protocols internationally, resulting in reductions in the length of hospital stays. These trials demonstrated that applying the ERAS principles could meaningfully impact daily clinical practice (8, 23).

A series of clinical trials followed, showing the effectiveness of ERAS. This culminated in a 2010 meta-analysis of six randomized controlled trials, which showed significant reductions in postoperative complications and the length of hospital stay by an average of 2.5 days (24).

The next challenge was assessing the implementation of ERAS on a broader scale. The Dutch Institute for Health Care Improvement conducted a clinical trial enrolling 33 hospitals that implemented ERAS protocols for elective colonic surgeries. The results showed a decrease in the length of hospital stay (25). However, adherence to ERAS elements in the postoperative phase was low at 56%, compared to 80% and 92% in the pre-and intraoperative phases, respectively (25).

However, protocol adherence has been identified as a key determinant of the effectiveness of the ERAS pathway. In their first meta-analysis of randomized studies in colorectal surgery, Gustafsson et al. have shown that higher protocol compliance rates correlated with better outcomes (26). Compliance above 70% has been shown to be effective in improving outcomes. In contrast, adherence below 50% was associated with poorer results (26). Subsequent trials have since reinforced the correlation between adherence and efficacy of ERAS protocols with improvements in postoperative complication rates, symptom burden, and readmission rates (27, 28).

In 2010, the ERAS® Study Group evolved into the ERAS® Society, which was formed as a non-profit medical society based in Sweden. The goal was to expand their efforts beyond research and education to include the implementation of the ERAS protocols (8). The ERAS® Interactive Audit System (EIAS), a cloud-based IT system, was also introduced. EIAS represents a database to collect data, monitor protocol adherence, support implementation, serve as a quality registry, and provide a basis for ongoing research (8, 21).

Since then, the ERAS® Society has continuously expanded its outreach internationally and across surgical subspecialties. It has developed several guidelines for multiple surgical specialties and procedures, including guidelines for gynecology and gynecologic oncology (7–9) (Figure 6.2).

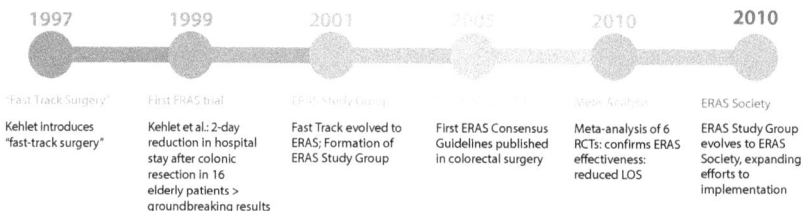

1997	1999	2001		2010	2010
"Fast Track Surgery"	First ERAS trial	ERAS Study Group		Meta-Analysis	ERAS Society
Kehlet introduces "fast-track surgery"	Kehlet et al.: 2-day reduction in hospital stay after colonic resection in 16 elderly patients > groundbreaking results	Fast Track evolved to ERAS; Formation of ERAS Study Group	First ERAS Consensus Guidelines published in colorectal surgery	Meta-analysis of 6 RCTs: confirms ERAS effectiveness: reduced LOS	ERAS Study Group evolves to ERAS Society, expanding efforts to implementation

FIGURE 6.2   ERAS milestones toward its application in gynecologic oncology.

6.4 ADOPTION OF ERAS IN GYNECOLOGIC ONCOLOGY: FIRST CLINICAL TRIALS AND GUIDELINE INTRODUCTION

The adoption of ERAS in gynecologic oncology was incremental but significant (18). The first prospective trial of ERAS in ovarian cancer patients was performed by Marx in 2006 (29) (Figure 6.3). In this trial, ten ERAS items were adapted from the colorectal guidelines and were implemented in 69 ovarian cancer patients. The results showed reductions in hospital stay length and severe postoperative morbidity (29).

Building on these initial findings, the 2008 trial by Gerardi et al. laid the foundation for the feasibility of ERAS protocols in patients with ovarian cancer (18, 30). The trial evaluated the effect of two ERAS items: early oral intake and early removal of the nasogastric tube, in ovarian cancer patients undergoing primary cytoreductive surgery with colorectal anastomosis. In this study of 19 patients, a reduction in the length of hospital stay and healthcare costs could be observed (30).

In 2013, Kalogera et al. expanded ERAS implementation to a broader cohort of patients undergoing various gynecologic procedures (31). Eleven ERAS items were implemented for 81 patients undergoing cytoreduction (e.g., bowel resection, splenectomy, diaphragm resection), 84 patients undergoing staging surgeries (e.g., hysterectomy, omentectomy, lymphadenectomy), and

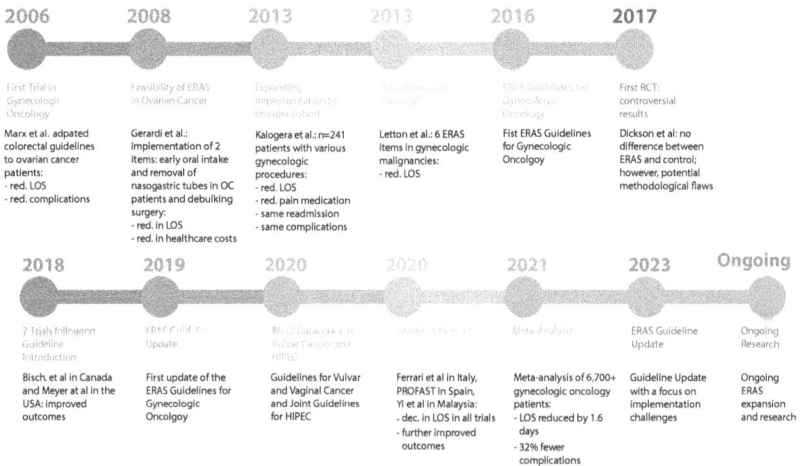

FIGURE 6.3   Evolution of ERAS in gynecologic oncology.

76 patients undergoing vaginal surgery. Among the total of 241 patients, the study showed significant improvements across several outcome parameters: a reduction in the length of hospital stay by four days, a reduction in healthcare costs, and a 65% reduction in patient-administered anesthesia in the cytoreduction group, as well as an overall reduction in the opioid use of 80%. Importantly, there was no increase in the complication- or readmission- rates, suggesting that ERAS is effective without compromising quality of care (31).

Another 2013 study by Letton et al., conducted in the UK, analyzed the effects of six ERAS items as part of an "integrated care pathway" in 52 patients undergoing abdominal or pelvic surgery for suspected or confirmed gynecologic malignancy. The study showed a moderate, though not statistically significant, reduction in hospital stay (32).

While early studies showed encouraging outcomes, a standardized ERAS protocol for gynecologic oncology had not yet been established. To standardize protocols, the first ERAS guidelines for gynecologic oncology, focusing on abdominal surgery, were published in 2016 and first updated in 2019 (7, 9). These guidelines drew upon existing evidence in gynecologic surgery, extrapolated data of the component evidence, and high-quality data from other surgical specialties, particularly colorectal surgery (18).

Gynecologic oncology includes a heterogeneous spectrum of patients and a broad scope of surgical procedures, spanning from minor local excisions for vulvar cancer to extensive operations like pelvic exenteration in advanced cancer or local recurrence. Therefore, separate guidelines for vulvar and vaginal cancers were released in 2020 (33). Although data remain limited due to the rarity of these procedures, ERAS principles from related surgical fields have guided the perioperative management in this particular patient cohort (18). In the same year, collaborative guidelines for cytoreductive surgery and hyperthermic intraperitoneal chemotherapy (HIPEC) in gynecologic and gastrointestinal oncology were also published (34).

6.5 FURTHER CLINICAL TRIALS FOLLOWING THE ERAS GUIDELINE INTRODUCTION AND EXPANDING IMPLEMENTATION

After the introduction of the ERAS guidelines, more clinical trials were performed to further assess their impact (18).

In 2018, two prospective cohort trials were published: one by Bisch et al. across a multicenter healthcare system in Canada and another by Meyer et al.

in the US. Both demonstrated improved outcomes in patients undergoing gynecologic oncologic surgeries (35, 36).

In the study by Bisch et al., 367 ERAS patients were compared with a historical control group of 152. Results included a 31% reduction in the length of hospital stay, a 6% reduction in postoperative complications, and decreased healthcare costs per patient (35).

In the study by Meyer et al., 553 ERAS patients were compared to a historical control group of 74 patients, showing a reduction in opioid use and patient-reported fatigue without an increase in reported pain (36).

The first prospective randomized trial in patients with gynecologic malignancies was performed in 2017 by Dickson et al., implementing nine ERAS items for 51 patients undergoing laparotomy compared to 51 control patients. The study found no differences between both arms (37). The publication of this trial led to controversies regarding the effectiveness of ERAS in gynecologic oncology. However, other researchers and proponents of ERAS highlighted methodological flaws in this trial (38). Among the methodological considerations were the omission of essential ERAS items, recommended by the International ERAS Society Guidelines, and a lack of reporting on protocol adherence, a major determinant of the success of ERAS (26, 37).

Subsequent randomized controlled trials followed in 2020. Ferrari et al. conducted a study in Italy with 83 ERAS patients and 85 controls undergoing surgery for suspected or confirmed gynecologic malignancy (39). Results showed a two-day reduction in the length of hospital stay, a 15% decrease in postoperative complications, and improved patient satisfaction (39).

Similarly, the prospective randomized controlled trial PROFAST in Spain was also conducted in 2020 (40). This trial, for patients with epithelial ovarian cancer undergoing primary-, secondary-, or interval-debulking surgery, randomized 49 patients to the ERAS group and 50 patients to the control group. The trial showed a two-day decrease in the length of hospital stay from nine to seven days (40).

Yi et al. conducted another prospective trial in Malaysia, implementing 12 ERAS items, with a focus on preoperative protein-infused carbohydrate loading, postoperative early feeding, and return to solid foods. Sixty-two ERAS patients were compared to 56 patients receiving standard care. The results showed a significant decrease in length of hospital stay and hospital readmission rates (41).

During the next 15 years following Marx et al.'s initial publication, a total of 31 comparative studies on ERAS in gynecologic oncology surgery were conducted. In 2021, Bisch et al. published a systematic review and meta-analysis, synthesizing these trials to present a comprehensive global overview of ERAS's effectiveness in gynecologic oncology surgery (42).

The meta-analysis included data from over 6,700 patients and assessed the impact of ERAS in gynecologic oncology surgery. The study reported that ERAS protocols were associated with an average reduction in hospital length of stay by 1.6 days, a 32% decrease in complication rates, and a 20% reduction in hospital readmissions. Additionally, cost analysis indicated an average saving of 2,129 USD per patient (42).

The analysis also examined specific complications and found improvements in respiratory, gastrointestinal, and renal outcomes. A major concern after the rise of ERAS protocols was the risk of anastomotic leaks following bowel resection. This rare complication was also evaluated in a subset of 1,195 patients, with pooled data showing no increased odds of anastomotic leaks following ERAS implementation (OR 0.93, 95% CI 0.35–2.53). Furthermore, the study found no difference in 30-day postoperative mortality rates between ERAS and standard care (42).

These findings further support the effectiveness and safety of ERAS protocols in gynecologic oncology surgery.

However, wide-scale ERAS implementation and protocol adherence remains a challenge. Due to the importance of adherence to ERAS protocols as a critical factor for influencing outcomes, attention has expanded to understanding and addressing the real-world challenges and barriers of ERAS implementation. This led to the publication of updated ERAS guidelines in 2023 with a focus on strategies to improve compliance and overcome obstacles to implementation (43).

6.6 PATIENT CONSIDERATIONS IN GYNECOLOGIC ONCOLOGY

Certain considerations are involved in gynecologic oncologic patients, a heterogeneous population that spans young individuals in good health to those who are severely frail with various comorbidities. The scope of surgical intervention is equally broad, ranging from minor local excision to complex operations, such as cytoreductive surgery or pelvic exenteration (18).

With an aging global population, the number of cancer diagnoses continues to rise, and advancing age and frailty have become central aspects of treatment planning (1, 11). These considerations are critical in deciding between treatment strategies, such as primary debulking surgery versus neoadjuvant chemotherapy, and guiding perioperative management strategies, particularly in the pre-treatment phase (44). Chronological age is insufficient; biological age, functional reserve, and comorbidities must be considered to personalize treatment strategies for the individual patient (11, 18, 44).

Patients with ovarian cancer often face preoperative challenges that can significantly impact surgical outcomes and the effectiveness of cancer treatment (18). They often present with a significant disease burden and ascites, which are frequently associated with malnutrition, hypalbuminemia, and sarcopenia (18, 45). These symptoms are often linked to cancer-related cachexia and bowel dysfunction, further aggravating malnutrition, muscle loss, and sarcopenia. In addition, psychosocial factors such as anxiety and reduced quality of life have been associated with worse postoperative outcomes (46).

Notably, many of these risk factors contributing to severe postoperative complications can be identified and potentially modified prior to surgery, presenting an opportunity for prehabilitation (18, 47, 48).

By addressing nutritional deficits, enhancing physical condition, supporting mental health, and improving general health status, prehabilitation offers a proactive approach to preparing patients for the demands of surgery. This, in turn, supports recovery and improves the overall care of patients with ovarian cancer.

6.7 HISTORICAL DEVELOPMENT AND CONCEPT OF PREHABILITATION

The period between a cancer diagnosis and the initiation of treatment presents a valuable opportunity to prepare patients for the upcoming stress of cancer treatment.

Prehabilitation refers to the proactive enhancement of a patient's functional capacity prior to a medical intervention, such as surgery (49, 50). While there is no universally accepted definition or standardized model, multimodal prehabilitation seems to be the most efficient and has gained recognition in recent years (9, 50). These programs aim to improve patients' general health and resilience by using multimodal approaches, targeting key areas such as physical fitness, nutrition status, and mental health before a medical intervention, improving patients' ability to withstand and recover from the upcoming procedure (50).

The concept of prehabilitation has evolved over several decades, its roots dating back to the mid–20th century. The term "prehabilitation" first appeared in the *British Medical Journal* in 1946, describing a program during the Second World War to prepare military recruits who were initially deemed unfit for service due to poor health (51). Over two months, recruits underwent a structured program, including physical training, nutritional support, and education. Over 85% of the 12,000 participants were successfully transformed into service-ready recruits (50, 51).

In the late 1980s, prehabilitation re-emerged within sports medicine, where it was used to prevent injuries in athletes (50).

By the late 1990s and early 2000s, the concept of prehabilitation was introduced into elective surgical care to improve postoperative outcomes (52).

In 1997, Weiner et al. investigated the effect of inspiratory muscle training in 17 patients before lung resection, aiming to improve postoperative pulmonary function. Compared to 15 control patients, those in the intervention group showed improved inspiratory muscle strength and pulmonary function post-surgery (53).

In 1999, Arthur et al. explored a prehabilitation intervention in patients awaiting coronary artery bypass graft surgery by actively utilizing the preoperative waiting period of at least 10 weeks. The intervention consisted of an exercise program twice weekly, patient education, and monthly telephone follow-ups. The intervention group showed a one-day reduction in the length of hospital stay and improved quality of life during the waiting period (54).

Prehabilitation was also explored in orthopedic surgery, initiated before knee arthroplasty. A case report in 2007 described two female patients completing a four-week prehabilitation program focused on strength and range of motion versus standard care. The participants showed improved physical outcomes and reduced postoperative pain (55).

In 2010, Nielsen et al. investigated the impact of a combined prehabilitation and early rehabilitation protocol in 28 patients undergoing lumbar spinal surgery versus 30 control patients. The prehabilitation intervention was two months long and consisted of an intensive exercise program, improved pain management, and a preoperative protein drink. Postoperatively, the intervention continued with early and intensified mobilization, protein supplementation, and optimized analgesia using epidurals. Compared to the control patients, those in the intervention group showed improved physical function at the time of surgery, earlier achievement of recovery milestones, and reduced length of hospital stay. Furthermore, patient satisfaction was significantly higher. There were no differences in postoperative complications, pain, or quality of life in the two groups (56).

6.8 PREHABILITATION IN ONCOLOGIC SURGICAL PATIENTS

By 2010, prehabilitation was used in oncological surgical care. Similarly to ERAS, prehabilitation in cancer surgery was first introduced for patients with colorectal cancer (57, 58).

In 2010, Carli et al. conducted a randomized controlled trial of prehabilitation in colorectal surgery (58). The intervention consisted of an exercise program averaging 54 days. Fifty-eight patients were randomized to a group performing biking and strength training, while 54 were assigned to a simpler protocol of walking and breathing exercises. There were no differences in walking capacity, although patients assigned to the easier walking/breathing group showed greater relative improvement in walking capacity (47% versus 22%). However, overall adherence to the intervention was low (58).

Following up on this trial, the same research group went on to explore the effects of a trimodal prehabilitation program, adding nutritional counseling with protein supplements and anxiety-reduction strategies to the pre-existing moderate physical exercise intervention for patients undergoing colorectal cancer resection (57). Forty-two patients received the prehabilitation intervention, which lasted 33 days on average, compared with 45 control patients who received standard care. Patients in the intervention group demonstrated better walking capacity after both the prehabilitation period and surgery. Moreover, 80% of patients in the intervention group had recovered by eight weeks postoperatively, compared to only 40% in the control group (57).

Subsequent trials extended the application of prehabilitation to patients with lung and esophageal cancers (59, 60). In lung cancer patients undergoing operative resection, strength and endurance training led to improvements in preoperative functional capacity and reduced respiratory morbidity (47). Similarly, Inoue et al. found that intensive respiratory (pre)- rehabilitation reduced postoperative pulmonary complications in patients undergoing esophagectomy for esophageal cancer (60).

6.9 PREHABILITATION IN GYNECOLOGIC ONCOLOGY

In gynecologic oncology, the integration of prehabilitation is an emerging area of clinical research, with several trials currently underway.

One of the earliest case reports was published in 2012 by Carli et al. (61). It was a report of an 88-year-old frail patient who underwent a three-week rehabilitation program prior to a robotic-assisted hysterectomy and showed improvements in exercise tolerance, cognitive function, and overall functional capacity (61).

Since then, interest has grown, and several trials have focused on patients with ovarian cancer. In 2022, Miralpeix et al. published results from a single-center pilot study evaluating a prehabilitation intervention involving 14 patients receiving neoadjuvant chemotherapy, compared to a historical control group of 15 patients managed with standard care, including ERAS. The prehabilitation protocol included a structured physical exercise program, nutritional counseling, and psychological support. Perioperative management was administered through the ERAS pathway in both arms. The intervention group showed improvements in protein levels, reduced need for blood transfusions, and fewer complications (62).

Recently, in June and October 2024, two prospective single-center trials were published for patients with ovarian cancer before debulking surgery (63, 64).

Zebalski et al. evaluated a multimodal prehabilitation program in Poland, which consisted of physical fitness, nutrition, psychological support, smoking- and alcohol cessation, and medical optimization, all integrated within the ERAS pathway. Thirty-six patients were enrolled in the intervention group and 34 in the control group. Patients in the intervention group demonstrated improved physical function (assessed by the 6-Minute Walk Test), and fewer complications compared to the control group (63).

Similarly, Sebio-Garcia et al. conducted a trial in Spain. The group investigated the effects of a prehabilitation intervention consisting of medical optimization, an exercise program, nutrition counseling, and psychological support for patients with advanced ovarian cancer undergoing primary or interval debulking surgery. Of the 62 patients referred to the prehabilitation program, 35 completed the preoperative assessment. Significant improvements were observed in the functional capacity (assessed by the 6-Minute Walk Test and Sit-to-Stand Test). Furthermore, there was an improvement in the overall Hospital Anxiety and Depression Scale (HADS) score and a decrease in depression in anxiety (64).

Currently, two prospective multicenter clinical trials are evaluating multimodal prehabilitation, integrating physical, nutritional, and psychological components alongside ERAS pathways, with the primary outcome of reducing postoperative complications (65, 66).

KORE-INNOVATION is a prospective, multicenter, controlled interventional study in Germany that is looking at the implementation and evaluation of a personalized trimodal prehabilitation program consisting of a physical fitness, nutrition, mental health, and empowerment intervention in combination with the ERAS pathway. The primary outcome is the rate of serious postoperative complications within 30 days post-surgery. Secondary outcomes include length of hospital stay, time to recovery, and quality-of-life measures (66).

The SOPHIE trial in Spain aims to assess whether a multimodal prehabilitation program can reduce postoperative complications in patients undergoing cytoreductive surgery for advanced ovarian cancer within an ERAS framework. The primary endpoint is the rate of postoperative complications, measured by the Comprehensive Complication Index (CCI). Secondary outcomes include length of hospital stay and time to initiation of adjuvant therapy (67).

Among ongoing trials, two studies with published protocols are specifically investigating prehabilitation during neoadjuvant chemotherapy (NACT) in ovarian cancer patients (68, 69).

The TRAINING-Ovary 01 trial, conducted at seven French comprehensive cancer centers, is investigating the effects of a home-based, patient-tailored physical activity program during neoadjuvant chemotherapy up until surgery. The primary outcome is cardiovascular fitness measured by the difference in maximum oxygen capacity (VO2max). Secondary outcomes include further physical outcome parameters, nutrition status, morbidity, and quality of life (68).

The PHOCUS trial is a randomized controlled study designed to evaluate the impact of a multimodal prehabilitation program consisting of physical fitness, dietary counseling, and a mental health intervention on patients undergoing surgery for gynecological cancers with a cohort of advanced stage (II–IV) ovarian cancer patients undergoing NACT. The goal is to improve physical function, measured by the 6-Minute-Walk Test (69).

Patient adherence is essential for the successful implementation and impact of prehabilitation. Some qualitative studies have explored patients' acceptance, experiences, and potential barriers to these programs (70).

In a qualitative study on gynecologic oncology surgery, a research group at Mayo Clinic interviewed 15 women with advanced ovarian cancer undergoing NACT in one-on-one semi-structured interviews. The interviews explored patients' views on exercise and physical activity during treatment. Many participants were highly motivated to engage in physical activity when recommended by their healthcare team, especially if they believed it could positively impact their treatment or chances of cure. However, several barriers were identified, including cancer- and treatment-related symptoms, limited access to programs, and social and mental challenges (70).

These early studies and ongoing trials show the exciting potential of prehabilitation and are laying the groundwork for its broader integration into standard perioperative care in gynecologic oncology. However, we are still in the early stages of prehabilitation strategies, and tangible results are missing. More research needs to be conducted to define prehabilitation, identify effective interventions and outcomes, and assess its feasibility and scalability.

Figure 6.4 provides the timeline of the evolution of prehabilitation in gynecologic oncology.

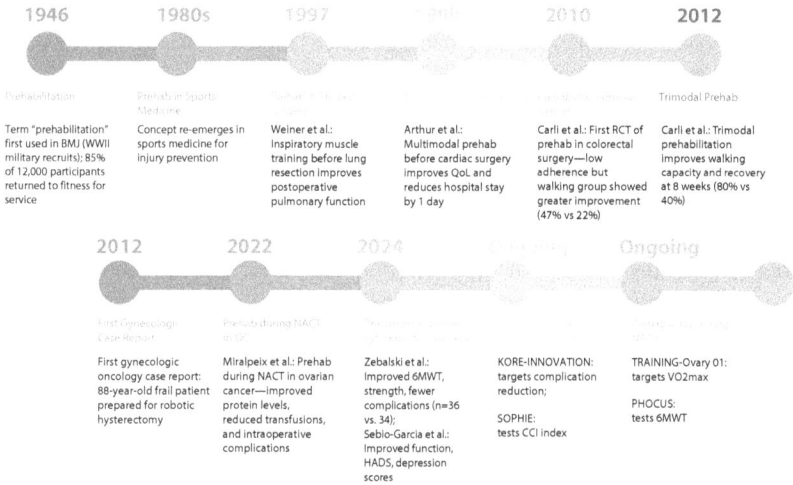

1946
Prehabilitation
Term "prehabilitation" first used in BMJ (WWII military recruits); 85% of 12,000 participants returned to fitness for service

1980s
Prehab in Sports Medicine
Concept re-emerges in sports medicine for injury prevention

1997
Weiner et al.: Inspiratory muscle training before lung resection improves postoperative pulmonary function

Arthur et al.: Multimodal prehab before cardiac surgery improves QoL and reduces hospital stay by 1 day

2010
Carli et al.: First RCT of prehab in colorectal surgery—low adherence but walking group showed greater improvement (47% vs 22%)

2012
Trimodal Prehab
Carli et al.: Trimodal prehabilitation improves walking capacity and recovery at 8 weeks (80% vs 40%)

2012
First Gynecologic Case Report
First gynecologic oncology case report: 88-year-old frail patient prepared for robotic hysterectomy

2022
Prehab during NACT in GO
Miralpeix et al.: Prehab during NACT in ovarian cancer—improved protein levels, reduced transfusions, and intraoperative complications

2024
Zebalski et al.: Improved 6MWT, strength, fewer complications (n=36 vs. 34); Sebio-Garcia et al.: Improved function, HADS, depression scores

KORE-INNOVATION: targets complication reduction;
SOPHIE: tests CCI index

Ongoing
TRAINING-Ovary 01: targets VO2max
PHOCUS: tests 6MWT

FIGURE 6.4 Timeline of the evolution of prehabilitation in gynecologic oncology.

6.10 CURRENT PRACTICE AND OUTLOOK

In recent years, ERAS protocols have continued to evolve within gynecologic oncology, incorporating technological and methodological advancements to optimize perioperative care.

ERAS protocols have demonstrated clear benefits and have significantly contributed to the standardization of perioperative care, leading to improved recovery outcomes and increased patient satisfaction. Nevertheless, challenges remain in achieving consistent implementation and protocol adherence across institutions, mainly due to resource variability, institutional infrastructure, and practitioner acceptance.

More recently, prehabilitation has emerged as a complementary strategy to ERAS, with several clinical trials underway. Prehabilitation aims to optimize patients' physical and psychological readiness for surgery by utilizing the window between diagnosis and treatment initiation. While ongoing research continues to refine best practices, current evidence supports a trimodal approach, combining physical fitness, nutritional optimization, and psychological support.

The evolution of perioperative care in gynecologic oncology reflects a broader shift from reactive, fragmented care to structured, interdisciplinary, and evidence-based approaches. The effectiveness of ERAS protocols depends on their consistent implementation and adherence tailored to the needs of diverse patient populations.

Future challenges will continue to be implementing and adhering to ERAS pathways across different healthcare systems and institutions and adapting protocol standards as research progresses. Furthermore, tailoring the protocols to specific surgical procedures and patient populations will be essential. The adaptation of ERAS protocols to resource-limited settings should be a main priority to ensure equitable access to high-quality care.

As for prehabilitation, a lot of questions currently remain unanswered. Further work is required to find a common definition of prehabilitation and establish a universal protocol in gynecologic oncology. Additionally, outcome measures need to be identified that clearly demonstrate its clinical benefit to patients and the feasibility of the intervention. Building on these results, scalability needs to be explored to support the integration of prehabilitation strategies into existing healthcare systems. Patient adherence to prehabilitation programs is another concern. In this context, remote and digitally supported programs may be a promising option to facilitate wider access and reduce disparities in care delivery, particularly in underserved settings.

The trajectory of ERAS and prehabilitation in gynecologic oncology reflects an ongoing evolution in perioperative care. Though continuous research is needed to refine the best practices further, the development of perioperative management shows the progressive shift toward a more comprehensive, patient-centric, personalized approach to care, encompassing the entire patient journey, spanning beyond the operating room.

REFERENCES

1. Armstrong DK et al. Ovarian cancer, Version 2.2020, NCCN clinical practice guidelines in oncology. *J Natl Compr Canc Netw.* 2021;*19*(2):191–226.
2. du Bois A et al. Role of surgical outcome as prognostic factor in advanced epithelial ovarian cancer: a combined exploratory analysis of 3 prospectively randomized phase 3 multicenter trials: by the Arbeitsgemeinschaft Gynaekologische Onkologie Studiengruppe Ovarialkarzinom (AGO-OVAR) and the Groupe d'Investigateurs Nationaux Pour les Etudes des Cancers de l'Ovaire (GINECO). *Cancer.* 2009;*115*(6):1234–44.
3. Fotopoulou C et al. European society of gynaecological oncology guidelines for the peri-operative management of advanced ovarian cancer patients undergoing debulking surgery. *Int J Gynecol Cancer.* 2021;*31*(9):1199–206.

4. Ljungqvist O et al. *Enhanced Recovery After Surgery. A Complete Guide to Optimizing Outcomes.* Springer Nature Switzerland AG, 2020.
5. Schwenk W et al. *Fast Track in der operativen Medizin.* Springer Medizin Verlag 2009.
6. Miralpeix E et al. A call for new standard of care in perioperative gynecologic oncology practice: Impact of enhanced recovery after surgery (ERAS) programs. *Gynecol Oncol.* 2016;*141*(2):371–8.
7. Nelson G et al. Guidelines for postoperative care in gynecologic/oncology surgery: Enhanced Recovery After Surgery (ERAS®) Society recommendations--Part II. *Gynecol Oncol.* 2016;*140*(2):323–32.
8. Ljungqvist O. Enhanced recovery after surgery and the ERAS® society. *J Pancreatol.* 2019;*2*(3):65–8.
9. Nelson G et al. Guidelines for perioperative care in gynecologic/oncology: Enhanced Recovery After Surgery (ERAS) Society recommendations–2019 update. *Int J Gynecol Cancer.* 2019;*29*(4):651–68.
10. Carli F et al. Effect of multimodal prehabilitation vs postoperative rehabilitation on 30-day postoperative complications for frail patients undergoing resection of colorectal cancer: A randomized clinical trial. *JAMA Surg.* 2020;*155*(3):233–42.
11. Inci MG et al. Can fried frailty score predict postoperative morbidity and mortality in gynecologic cancer surgery? Results of a prospective study. *J Geriatr Oncol.* 2021;*12*(3):428–33.
12. Fukushima R, Kaibori M. *Enhanced Recovery after Surgery.* Springer Nature Singapore 2018.
13. Finnerty CC et al. The surgically induced stress response. *JPEN J Parenter Enteral Nutr.* 2013;*37*(5 Suppl):21S–9S.
14. Minig L et al. Early oral versus "traditional" postoperative feeding in gynecologic oncology patients undergoing intestinal resection: a randomized controlled trial. *Ann Surg Oncol.* 2009;*16*(6):1660–8.
15. Carli F et al. Epidural analgesia enhances functional exercise capacity and health-related quality of life after colonic surgery: results of a randomized trial. *Anesthesiology.* 2002;*97*(3):540–9.
16. Ljungqvist O et al. The history of enhanced recovery after surgery and the ERAS society. *J Laparoendosc Adv Surg Tech A.* 2017;*27*(9):860–2.
17. Kehlet H. Multimodal approach to control postoperative pathophysiology and rehabilitation. *Br J Anaesth.* 1997;*78*(5):606–17.
18. Nelson G, et al. *The ERAS Society Handbook for Obstetrics & Gynecology.* Academic Press; Elsevier Inc. 2022.
19. Gordon TA et al. The effects of regionalization on cost and outcome for one general high-risk surgical procedure. *Ann Surg.* 1995;*221*(1):43–9.
20. Kehlet H et al. Hospital stay of 2 days after open sigmoidectomy with a multimodal rehabilitation programme. *Br J Surg.* 1999;*86*(2):227–30.
21. Golder HJ, Papalois V. Enhanced recovery after surgery: History, key advancements and developments in transplant surgery. *J Clin Med.* 2021;*10*(8):1–14.
22. Fearon KC et al. Enhanced recovery after surgery: a consensus review of clinical care for patients undergoing colonic resection. *Clin Nutr.* 2005;*24*(3):466–77.
23. Lassen K et al. Patterns in current perioperative practice: survey of colorectal surgeons in five northern European countries. *BMJ.* 2005;*330*(7505):1420–1.

24. Varadhan KK et al. The enhanced recovery after surgery (ERAS) pathway for patients undergoing major elective open colorectal surgery: a meta-analysis of randomized controlled trials. *Clin Nutr.* 2010;*29*(4):434–40.
25. Gillissen F et al. Structured synchronous implementation of an enhanced recovery program in elective colonic surgery in 33 hospitals in The Netherlands. *World J Surg.* 2013;*37*(5):1082–93.
26. Gustafsson UO et al. Adherence to the enhanced recovery after surgery protocol and outcomes after colorectal cancer surgery. *Arch Surg.* 2011;*146*(5):571–7.
27. Gustafsson UO et al. Adherence to the ERAS protocol is Associated with 5-Year Survival After Colorectal Cancer Surgery: A Retrospective Cohort Study. *World J Surg.* 2016;*40*(7):1741–7.
28. The impact of enhanced recovery protocol compliance on elective colorectal cancer resection: Results from an international registry. *Ann Surg.* 2015;*261*(6):1153–9.
29. Marx C et al. The effect of accelerated rehabilitation on recovery after surgery for ovarian malignancy. *Acta Obstet Gynecol Scand.* 2006;*85*(4):488–92.
30. Gerardi MA et al. A clinical pathway for patients undergoing primary cytoreductive surgery with rectosigmoid colectomy for advanced ovarian and primary peritoneal cancers. *Gynecol Oncol.* 2008;*108*(2):282–6.
31. Kalogera E et al. Enhanced recovery in gynecologic surgery. *Obstet Gynecol.* 2013;*122*(2 Pt 1):319–28.
32. Letton C et al. Does an enhanced recovery integrated care pathway (ICP) encourage adherence to prescribing guidelines, accelerate postoperative recovery and reduce the length of stay for gynaecological oncology patients? *J Obstet Gynaecol.* 2013;*33*(3):296–7.
33. Altman AD et al. Guidelines for vulvar and vaginal surgery: Enhanced recovery after surgery society recommendations. *Am J Obstet Gynecol.* 2020;*223*(4):475–85.
34. Hübner M et al. Guidelines for perioperative care in cytoreductive surgery (CRS) with or without hyperthermic IntraPEritoneal chemotherapy (HIPEC): Enhanced recovery after surgery (ERAS®) Society Recommendations - Part I: Preoperative and intraoperative management. *Eur J Surg Oncol.* 2020;*46*(12):2292–310.
35. Bisch SP et al. Enhanced recovery after surgery (ERAS) in gynecologic oncology: System-wide implementation and audit leads to improved value and patient outcomes. *Gynecol Oncol.* 2018;*151*(1):117–23.
36. Meyer LA et al. Effect of an enhanced recovery after surgery program on opioid use and patient-reported outcomes. *Obstet Gynecol.* 2018;*132*(2):281–90.
37. Dickson EL et al. Enhanced recovery program and length of stay after laparotomy on a gynecologic oncology service: A randomized controlled trial. *Obstet Gynecol.* 2017;*129*(2):355–62.
38. Nelson G et al. Enhanced recovery program and length of stay after laparotomy on a gynecologic oncology service: A randomized controlled trial. *Obstet Gynecol.* 2017;*129*(6):1139.
39. Ferrari F et al. Validation of an enhanced recovery after surgery protocol in gynecologic surgery: an Italian randomized study, a response. *Am J Obstet Gynecol.* 2021;*224*(3):336–7.
40. Sánchez-Iglesias JL et al. PROFAST: A randomised trial implementing enhanced recovery after surgery for highcomplexity advanced ovarian cancer surgery. *Eur J Cancer.* 2020;*136*:149–58.

41. Yi HC et al. Impact of enhanced recovery after surgery with preoperative whey protein-infused carbohydrate loading and postoperative early oral feeding among surgical gynecologic cancer patients: An open-labelled randomized controlled trial. *Nutrients.* 2020;*12*(1).

42. Bisch SP et al. Outcomes of enhanced recovery after surgery (ERAS) in gynecologic oncology - A systematic review and meta-analysis. *Gynecol Oncol.* 2021; *161*(1):46–55.

43. Nelson G et al. Enhanced recovery after surgery (ERAS®) society guidelines for gynecologic oncology: Addressing implementation challenges - 2023 update. *Gynecol Oncol.* 2023;*173*:58–67.

44. Fadadu PP et al. Patients triaged to neoadjuvant chemotherapy have higher rates of sarcopenia: An opportunity for prehabilitation. *Gynecol Oncol.* 2021; *160*(1):40–4.

45. Sehouli J et al. Effects of sarcopenia and malnutrition on morbidity and mortality in gynecologic cancer surgery: results of a prospective study. *J Cachexia Sarcopenia Muscle.* 2021;*12*(2):393–402.

46. Inci MG et al. Patient-reported outcomes (PROs) and health-related quality of life (HR-QOL) in patients with ovarian cancer: what is different compared to healthy women? *Cancers (Basel).* 2021;*13*(4):1–11.

47. Kalogera E, Dowdy S. Prehabilitation: enhancing the enhanced recovery after surgery pathway. *Int J Gynecol Cancer.* 2019;*29*:1233–4.

48. Kumar A et al. Risk-prediction model of severe postoperative complications after primary debulking surgery for advanced ovarian cancer. *Gynecol Oncol.* 2016;*140*(1):15–21.

49. ACS, *Clinical Congress News* [Internet], 2024: www.facs.org/for-medical-professionals/news-publications/news-and-articles/cc2024-news/surgeons-highlight-the-growing-importance-of-prehabilitation/

50. Banugo P. Prehabilitation. *BJA Education.* 2017;*17*(12):401–5.

51. Prehabilitation, rehabilitation, and revocation in the Army. *Br Med J.* 1946; *1*:192–7.

52. Fleurent-Grégoire C et al. Towards a common definition of surgical prehabilitation: a scoping review of randomised trials. *Br J Anaesth.* 2024;*133*(2):305–15.

53. Weiner P et al. The effect of incentive spirometry and inspiratory muscle training on pulmonary function after lung resection. *J Thorac Cardiovasc Surg.* 1997;*113*(3):552–7.

54. Arthur HM et al. Effect of a preoperative intervention on preoperative and postoperative outcomes in low-risk patients awaiting elective coronary artery bypass graft surgery. A randomized, controlled trial. *Ann Intern Med.* 2000; *133*(4):253–62.

55. Jaggers JR et al. Prehabilitation before knee arthroplasty increases postsurgical function: a case study. *J Strength Cond Res.* 2007;*21*(2):632–4.

56. Nielsen PR et al. Prehabilitation and early rehabilitation after spinal surgery: randomized clinical trial. *Clin Rehabil.* 2010;*24*(2):137–48.

57. Li C et al. Impact of a trimodal prehabilitation program on functional recovery after colorectal cancer surgery: a pilot study. *Surg Endosc.* 2013;*27*(4):1072–82.

58. Carli F et al. Randomized clinical trial of prehabilitation in colorectal surgery. *Br J Surg.* 2010;*97*(8):1187–97.

59. Morano MT et al. Preoperative pulmonary rehabilitation versus chest physical therapy in patients undergoing lung cancer resection: a pilot randomized controlled trial. *Arch Phys Med Rehabil.* 2013;*94*(1):53–8.
60. Inoue J et al. Prevention of postoperative pulmonary complications through intensive preoperative respiratory rehabilitation in patients with esophageal cancer. *Dis Esophagus.* 2013;*26*(1):68–74.
61. Carli F et al. Prehabilitation to enhance postoperative recovery for an octogenarian following robotic-assisted hysterectomy with endometrial cancer. *Can J Anaesth.* 2012;*59*(8):779–84.
62. Miralpeix E et al. Impact of prehabilitation during neoadjuvant chemotherapy and interval cytoreductive surgery on ovarian cancer patients: a pilot study. *World J Surg Oncol.* 2022;*20*(1):46.
63. Zębalski MA et al. LUNA EMG as a marker of adherence to prehabilitation programs and its effect on postoperative outcomes among patients undergoing cytoreductive surgery for ovarian cancer and suspected ovarian tumors. *Cancers (Basel).* 2024;*16*(14).
64. Sebio-Garcia R et al. Multimodal prehabilitation improves functional capacity in patients with advanced ovarian cancer undergoing cytoreductive surgery. *Int J Gynecol Cancer.* 2024. https://doi.org/10.1136/ijgc-2024-005686
65. Díaz-Feijoo B et al. A multimodal prehabilitation program for the reduction of post-operative complications after surgery in advanced ovarian cancer under an ERAS pathway: a randomized multicenter trial (SOPHIE). *Int J Gynecol Cancer.* 2022. https://doi.org/10.1136/ijgc-2022-003652
66. Inci MG et al. The KORE-INNOVATION trial, a prospective controlled multi-site clinical study to implement and assess the effects of an innovative peri-operative care pathway for patients with ovarian cancer: rationale, methods and trial design. *Int J Gynecol Cancer.* 2023. https://doi.org/10.1136/ijgc-2023-004531
67. Díaz-Feijoo B et al. A multimodal prehabilitation program for the reduction of post-operative complications after surgery in advanced ovarian cancer under an ERAS pathway: a randomized multicenter trial (SOPHIE). *Int J Gynecol Cancer.* 2022;*32*(11):1463–8.
68. Lambaudie E et al. TRAINING-Ovary 01 (connecTed pRehabiliAtIoN pelvIc caNcer surGery): multicenter randomized study comparing neoadjuvant chemotherapy for patients managed for ovarian cancer with or without a connected pre-habilitation program. *Int J Gynecol Cancer.* 2021;*31*(6):920–4.
69. Mayer A, Cibula D. Optimizing prehabilitation in gynecologic malignancies: Improving acceptance, overcoming barriers, and managing program complexity. *Eur J Surg Oncol.* 2024;*50*(12):108739.
70. Polen-De C et al. Advanced ovarian cancer patients identify opportunities for prehabilitation: A qualitative study. *Gynecol Oncol Rep.* 2021;*36*:100731.

Index

Pages in *italics* refer to figures.

A

ADCC, *see* antibody dependent cell mediated cytotoxicity
adoptive cell therapy, 90
3-amino-benzamides, 70
antibody dependent cell mediated cytotoxicity (ADCC), 3
antibody-drug conjugates (ADC), 93–4
antigen-autoantibody complexes, 15
Arbeitsgemeinschaft Gynäkologische Onkologie (AGO) score, 37–8
atezolizumab, 89
ATHENA-COMBO trial, 75
Athenaeus, 26
autoantibodies, 14–5

B

BCG (*Bacillus calmette* Guerin), 2–3
benzamides, 70
bevacizumab, 31–2, 38–9, 89, 92
    durvalumab, 75, 95
    olaparib, 74–5, 95
    PARP inhibitors, 79, 95
biomarkers, 11
    detecting early-stage ovarian cancer, 12–7
    immunotherapy, 87–8
    metabolites, 16–7
    protein antigens, 12–4
biovectors, 92–3; *see also* vaccines
bispecific antibodies, 94–5
BRACAnalysis large rearrangement test (BART), 54–5
BRCA1, 10, 51–5, 57–9
BRCA2, 10, 52–5, 57–9

breast cancer, 50–1; *see also BRCA1*; *BRCA2*
breast cancer linkage consortium (BCLC), 51
Bridges, Calvin, 69
Broca, Pierre Paul, 48

C

CA72.4, 12–3
CA125 (Cancer Antigen 125), 2–4
    biomarkers, 12–7
    multi-cancer screening, 17
    single modality screening, 4
    two-stage strategies, 4–10
cancer
    as contagious, 47–8
    families with a high prevalence, 47
    genetics, 48–50
Cancer Antigen 125, *see* CA125 (Cancer Antigen 125)
CancerSEEK, 17
cancer vaccines, *see* vaccines
cell-free DNA (cfDNA), 16
chemotherapy
    adjuvant, 28, 30–3
    HIPEC, 31, 33, 41
    intraperitoneal (IP), 31
    neoadjuvant, 33–7, 39–40, 116
chimeric antigen receptor (CAR)-T cell, 86, 91
    CRISPR-Cas9, 96
    targets, 91
CHORUS trial, 34
circulating tumor DNA (ctDNA), 16
Coley, William, 85, 91
complementary DNA (cDNA), 52–3

123

Comprehensive Complication Index
    (CCI), 116
Corynebacterium parvum, 2–3
Crawford, Jane Todd, 27
CRISPR-Cas9, 96
cytoreduction/cytoreductive surgery, 101–3
    minimally invasive, 39–40
    neoadjuvant chemotherapy (NACT)
        vs., 33–7
    secondary, 37–9
cytotoxic T-lymphocyte-associated
    antigen 4 (CTLA-4), 86,
    89–90

D

dendritic cells (DC), 92
DESKTOP I, 37
DESKTOP II, 38
DESKTOP III, 38–9
DETECT-A study, 17
DNA
    cell-free (cfDNA), 16
    circulating tumor (ctDNA), 16
    complementary, 52–3
    methylation, 16
    mutations, 16
    repair systems, 69
durvalumab, 75

E

Eastern Cooperative Oncology Group
    (ECOG), 37
Enhanced Recovery after Surgery
    (ERAS), 102, 117–18
    clinical trials, 108–11
    concept, 103–4
    emergence, 104–7
    guidelines, 109
    milestones, *107*
    pathway, 103–4, *104*
ethyleneimine, 69–70

F

fast-track rehabilitation, 102; *see also*
    Enhanced Recovery after Surgery
    (ERAS)

G

Genetic Information Nondiscrimination
    Act (GINA), 55–6
genetics, 48–50
genetic testing
    discrimination, 55–6
    evolution, 53–5
Gompertzian growth model, 33
Griffiths, C. Thomas, 27–8
gynecologic oncology, 27
    ERAS, *see* Enhanced Recovery after
        Surgery (ERAS)
    prehabilitation, 114–16, *117*
Gynecologic Oncology Group (GOG), 28

H

HE4, 12–5
HIPEC (hyperthermic intraperitoneal
    chemotherapy), 31, 33, 41
homologous recombination deficiency
    (HRD), 89
Hospital Anxiety and Depression Scale
    (HADS) score, 115
Human Genome Project, 51
Huntington *(HTT)* gene, 50
Huntington's disease, 50
Hypoalbuminemia, 36

I

imaging, 17–8
IMagyn050 trial, 89
immune checkpoint inhibitors, 88–90
immune gene signatures, 87
immunosuppressive tumor
    microenvironment, 93
immunotherapy, 85–6
    antibody-drug conjugates (ADC),
        93–4
    biomarkers, 87–8
    bispecific antibodies, 94–5
    chemotherapy with, 88–9
    combination strategies, 95
    immune checkpoint inhibitors, 88–90
    major developments, timeline of, *86*
    novel approaches, 94
    pioneering studies, 96

radiation and, 96
   vaccines, 91–3
International ERAS Society Guidelines, 110
International Ovarian Tumor Analysis
   (IOTA), 18
intraperitoneal (IP) chemotherapy, 31
ipilimumab, 86, 90

J

Japan Clinical Oncology Group (JCOG),
   34–5
JAVELIN Ovarian 100 trial, 89
JAVELIN Ovarian 200, 89

K

KEYNOTE-028, 88
KORE-INNOVATION, 115

L

Li-Fraumeni syndrome, 10, 50
lymphadenectomy, 30
Lynch, Henry T., 49–50
Lynch syndrome, 50, 57

M

Mechanism of Mendelian Heredity
   (Morgan), 49
Meigs, Joe, 27
metabolites, 16–7
methylation of DNA, 16
MicroRNAs, 15
Six6-Minute-Walk Test, 116
MIRASOL trial, 94
mirvetuximab soravtansine-gynx
   (MIRV), 94
monoclonal antibodies (mAbs), 85–6, 93
mucin protein (MUC16), 3, 12
multi-cancer screening, 17
Myriad Genetics, 51–5

N

NACT, *see* neoadjuvant chemotherapy
NAD+, 69–70

National Cancer Institute, 50
National Comprehensive Cancer
   Network (NCCN), 8, 55
National Institutes of Health (NIH), 54
NCCN, *see* National Comprehensive
   Cancer Network
neoadjuvant chemotherapy (NACT),
   33–7, 39–40, 116
nicotinamide, 69–70
niraparib, 78
   first-line single-agent maintenance
      therapy, 73
   second-line maintenance therapy, 76–7
non-coding RNAs, 15; *see also*
   MicroRNAs
Normal Risk Ovarian Cancer Screening
   Study (NROSS) trial, 6, 7, 8–10,
   12, 14, 17–9

O

OC125 (125th promising clone), 3
olaparib, 70, 78
   bevacizumab and, 74–5
   clinical trials, 71–2
   FDA approval, 58–9, 72
   first-line maintenance combination
      theraoy, 74–5
   first-line single-agent maintenance,
      72–3
   germline *BRCA* mutations, 71–2
   second-line single-agent maintenance,
      76–7
Olvi-Vec, 93
oncolytic viruses, 92–3
oral contraceptive pills (OCP), 57
osteopontin (OPN), 13–4
ovarian cancer, 1–2; *see also BRCA1*;
   BRCA2
   care standard, 84–5
   death, leading cause of, 84
   heterogeneity, 93
   immunotherapy, *see* immunotherapy
   patient considerations, 111–12
   preoperative challenges, 112
   as a prevalent cancer, 84
   screening, *see* screening
OVERA, 4, 13

P

pegylated liposomal doxorubicin
　　(PLD), 89
pembrolizumab, 88–9
peptide vaccines, 92
perioperative care, 101–18
　　ERAS, *see* Enhanced Recovery after
　　　Surgery (ERAS)
　　prehabilitation, 102, 112–16
PET-CT imaging, 17–8
PHOCUS trial, 116
Photoacoustic imaging, 18
PLCO (Prostate, Lung, Colon, and
　　Ovary) Cancer Screening Trial, 4
poly (adenosine diphosphate-ribose)
　　polymerase (PARP) inhibitors,
　　68–79, 89, 95
　　discovery and development, *68*,
　　　69–71
　　DNA repair deficiency, 69
　　FDA approval, 68
　　immune checkpoint inhibitors, 75
　　late-line treatment, 78–9
　　niraparib, *see* niraparib
　　olaparib, *see* olaparib
　　rucaparib, *see* rucaparib
　　VEGF inhibitors, 74–5
　　voluntary withdrawal, 78–9
prehabilitation, 102, 112–16
　　colorectal surgery, 113–14
　　defined, 112
　　gynecologic oncology, 114–16, *117*
　　multicenter clinical trials,
　　　115–16
　　multimodal, 112
　　neoadjuvant chemotherapy
　　　(NACT), 116
　　patient adherence, 116
　　timeline (of evolution), *117*
programmed cell death protein 1
　　(PD-1), 86, 88
programmed death-ligand 1 (PD-L1),
　　86–9
protein antigens, 12–4

R

radiation
　　immunogenic cell death, 96
　　immunotherapy and, 96
Risk of Malignancy Algorithm (ROMA),
　　3, 13
risk of ovarian cancer algorithm (ROCA)
　　CA125 values, 5–9
　　ROCA2, 14, 19
　　screening trials, 6–9
risk-reducing surgery (RRS), 11
rituximab, 86
rucaparib, 70
　　first-line single-agent maintenance
　　　therapy, 73
　　second-line maintenance therapy, 77–8

S

Sanger sequencing, 53–4
SCORPION, 34–5
screening
　　biomarkers, 11–7
　　imaging, 17–8
　　improving initial stage, 11–7
　　multiple cancers, 17
　　two-stage strategies, 4–10
　　cost effectiveness, 10
　　mortality, 6–8, *8*, 9–10
　　stage shift, 9–10
　　women with high risk, 10–1
Serratia marcescens, 85, 91
SOPHIE trial, 115–16
Streptococcus pyogenes, 85, 91
Superconducting Quantum Interference
　　Detection (SQUID), 18
synthetic lethality, 69

T

temozolomide, 70
topotecan, 70
TP53, 10, 14–5
TRAINING-Ovary 01 trial, 116

transvaginal sonography (TVS), 2,
    4–11, 14, 17–8; *see also*
    screening
TRICARE insurance program, 56
tumor-infiltrating lymphocytes (TIL), 87,
    90–1
tumor mutational burden (TMB), 87

U

UKCTOCS (United Kingdom
    Collaborative Trial of Ovarian
    Cancer Screening), 6–10, 14, 17–9
UKFOCSS (UK Familial Ovarian Cancer
    Screening Study), 11

V

vaccines, 91–3
    biovectors, 92–3
    clinical efficacy, 93
    dendritic cell, 92
    peptide, 92
vascular endothelial growth factor
    (VEGF), 31
viruses
    oncolytic, 92–3

W

Warthin, Aldred Scott, 49
Wilms' Tumor 1 (WT1), 92

For Product Safety Concerns and Information please contact our EU
representative GPSR@taylorandfrancis.com
Taylor & Francis Verlag GmbH, Kaufingerstraße 24, 80331 München, Germany